Airways Obstruction

Duncan M. Geddes

MD, MRCP

Consultant Physician at the London Chest and Brompton
Hospitals, London

Published,
in association with
UPDATE PUBLICATIONS LTD., by

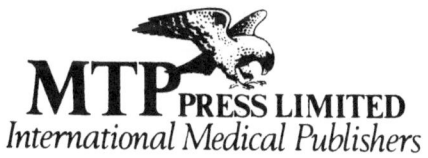

MTP **PRESS LIMITED**
International Medical Publishers

Published,
in association with
Update Publications Ltd., by

MTP Press Limited
Falcon House
Lancaster, England

ISBN-13: 978-94-009-8080-8   e-ISBN-13: 978-94-009-8078-5

DOI: 10.1007/ 978-94-009-8078-5

Contents

1. Mechanisms and Causes of Airflow Obstruction

Mechanisms

Airflow obstruction is characterized by reduced expiratory flow rates.

Expiration

During expiration, air flows from alveoli to the mouth because there is a pressure difference between them. The rate of airflow depends upon this pressure difference as well as the resistance to flow. The alveolar pressure is in part a property of the alveolar walls, while the resistance to airflow is a property of the airways. One must therefore look at both alveoli and airways to understand the mechanism of expiratory airflow limitation.

Alveoli (Figure 1)

The pressure driving expiratory airflow is the alveolar pressure. This comprises pressure applied to the alveoli from outside added to the elastic recoil of the alveolar walls. The pressure from outside is the positive intrapleural pressure generated by the expiratory muscles, while the recoil of the alveoli is due to their inherent elasticity. This elastic recoil is greatest when the lungs are fully inflated and diminishes during expiration as the lungs get smaller. The elasticity of the alveoli can be altered by disease: they are less elastic (more compliant) in emphysema and more elastic (less compliant) in pulmonary fibrosis. As well as affecting the alveolar pressure, this elasticity also exerts a pull on the airways, helping to hold them open.

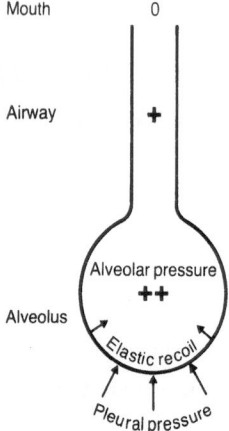

Figure 1. *Alveolar pressure = pleural pressure + elastic recoil.*

Airways

Resistance to airflow is related to the cross-sectional area of the airways. Any reduction in this area will increase resistance to airflow. This may occur in two ways:

1. Local narrowing of an airway, e.g. tracheal tumour.

2. Diffuse narrowing or obliteration of many airways, e.g. bronchoconstriction in asthma.

Interaction between Airways and Alveoli (Figure 2)

The floppy small airways will tend to collapse if pressure is exerted from outside. This outside pressure is the same intrapleural pressure as is applied to the alveoli during forced expiration. The airways do not collapse because of the elastic recoil of the alveoli. The alveoli hold the small airways open from the outside by radial traction on the airway walls and from the inside by generation of the alveolar pressure which is conducted down the airways. The radial traction depends both on the elasticity of the alveoli and on the degree of inflation of the lungs, so that airways collapse will

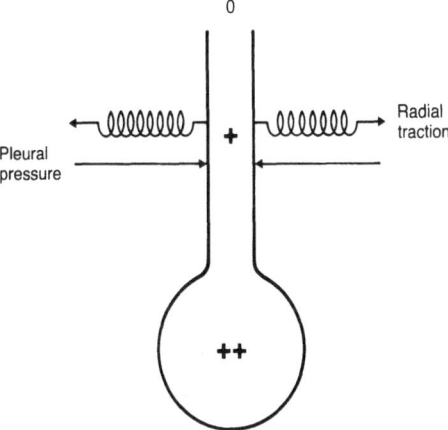

Figure 2. *Airway calibre depends on intraluminal pressure, radial traction and pleural pressure.*

tend to occur if the lungs are floppy (emphysema) and at the end of expiration when the alveoli are no longer distended (Figure 3). This leaves the residual volume behind the collapsed airways.

One important consequence of this expiratory airway narrowing and collapse is that flow rates for much of a forced expiration cannot be increased by greater expiratory effort. Any increased muscular effort will cancel itself out by narrowing airways as much as it increases alveolar pressure.

While all the airways contribute some resistance to airflow, flow rates are chiefly determined by the narrowest part of the bronchial tree. Normally this is the trachea since the total cross-sectional area of the airways increases dramatically as they branch, becoming very great in the last few generations before the alveoli (Figure 4). It follows that narrowing of the airways will have very different effects at different levels in the bronchial tree. A small tumour can drastically narrow the trachea and cause asphyxiation, while in the periphery of the lung, loss of many of the small airways will cause negligible increase in resistance to airflow.

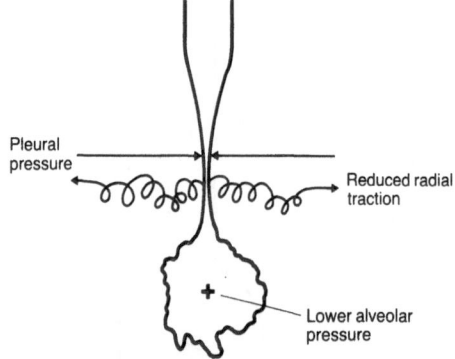

Figure 3. *Airways collapse in expiration as shrinking alveoli generate less elastic recoil and less radial traction.*

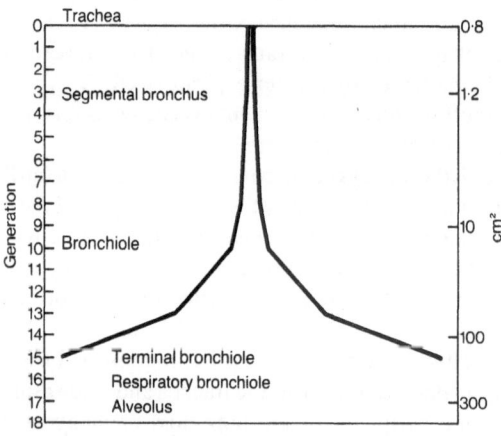

Figure 4. *Airway cross-sectional area increases peripherally.*

Inspiration (Figure 5)

The same arguments apply to inspiration with the important difference that the intrathoracic pressure is negative and this pulls open both alveoli and airways. This means that airways within the chest are actually widened by the muscular effort of inspiration and so resistance to airflow is diminished. For much of inspiration, flow rates are therefore higher than in forced expiration. While flow rates in expiration are largely independent of muscular effort, this is not the case in inspiration and so inspiratory flows are in part dependent on neuromuscular function.

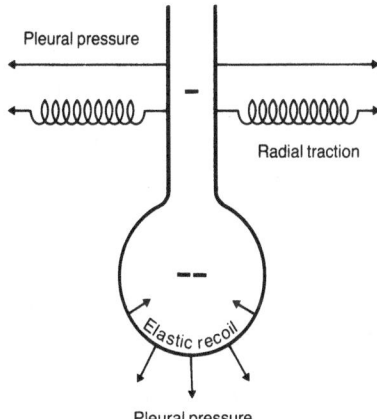

Figure 5. *Inspiratory airway widening (intrathoracic).*

Extrathoracic Airways

The upper parts of the trachea and larynx are outside the chest and so not affected by changes in intrapleural pressure. Changes in calibre with respiration are therefore opposite to the changes in airways within the chest. This is because the only pressure changes tending to alter the calibre of the trachea come from within the lumen. In expiration, intratracheal pressure is greater than atmospheric (so air flows towards the mouth), and in inspiration the pressure is less than atmospheric (so air flows from the mouth into the chest). This means that in expiration, the airway walls will be pushed out and the airway widened and in inspiration the airway will be narrowed. This is important since it allows intra- and extrathoracic causes of airflow obstruction to be differentiated by flow rates. Intrathoracic tumours will limit air-flow more in expiration than in inspiration, while extrathoracic tumours (or bilateral laryngeal palsy) will reduce airflow more in inspiration than in expiration (Figure 6).

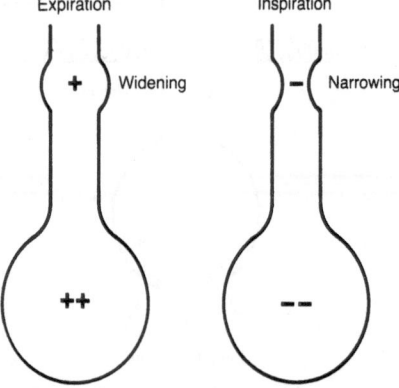

Figure 6. *Extrathoracic airway calibre is affected by intraluminal pressure only.*

Causes

These can conveniently be divided into local lesions which affect large airways and diffuse lesions affecting medium and small airways.

Large Airways

In the lumen:	Tumour, foreign body (e.g. peanut).
In the wall:	Tumour, stenosis, laryngeal palsy, defective cartilage.

Outside the wall: Lymph nodes, tumour.

These causes of airflow obstruction are relatively rare, and diagnosis is simple when the possibility of large airway obstruction is considered. As well as causing grossly abnormal lung function tests, the obstruction can be seen both radiographically and through a bronchoscope.

Small and Medium Airways

In the lumen:	Mucus, pus, oedema, fluid, plugs of mucus or fungi.
In the wall:	Mucous gland hypertrophy, muscle hypertrophy and spasm, inflammation (cells and oedema).

Outside the wall: Peribronchial inflammation and oedema, reduced radial traction, volume dependent airway collapse.

These causes of airflow obstruction are common. In any patient, many of these factors usually coexist and in particular, whenever medium and small airways are diffusely narrowed, airways will collapse earlier in expiration.

2. Assessment and Clinical Patterns

Airways obstruction can be diagnosed by clinical examination or by lung function testing. Both of these methods are crude and considerable damage to the small airways may occur before producing symptoms, abnormal signs or diagnostic changes in routine tests. When it comes to assessing the severity of the obstruction, clinical examination is unreliable and some form of lung function test must be used.

Assessment

Clinical Examination

Forced Expired Time

Airway obstruction within the chest will prolong expiration. This can be heard during routine auscultation. It is measured by timing the expiration of the vital capacity. The patient breathes in to full inspiration and then blows out to full expiration as fast as possible, while the examiner listens over the trachea with a stethoscope. The normal forced expired time is three seconds and in airways obstruction this increases to six seconds or more. The forced expired time is valueless in assessing the severity of the obstruction.

Wheeze

Wheezes are continuous musical noises which may be heard either through the chest wall or at the mouth. They are generated by oscillation of the airway walls during airflow and the pitch of the wheeze depends on the mechanical properties of the airway wall.

Wheezes are of limited value in diagnosis because:

1. All that wheezes is not asthma.

2. The worst obstruction does not wheeze, because the airflow is insufficient to make the airways oscillate.

Stridor is a loud wheeze produced by the upper airways. When it is loudest in inspiration the obstruction is likely to be in the extrathoracic trachea. A fixed monophonic wheeze suggests obstruction of a major airway, usually by a tumour.

Hyperinflation

A barrel chest is seen in chronic bronchitis and during an acute attack of asthma. This sign is only obvious when the obstruction is severe.

An acute asthmatic attack and the clinical assessment of respiratory failure are discussed in Chapters 6 and 8.

Lung Function Tests

All lung function test results are compared with the predicted normal value derived from the patient's age, sex and height.

Peak Expiratory Flow Rate (Peak Flow)

The peak flow is the maximum rate of airflow during a forced expiration. It depends on muscular effort, airways resistance, and the maintenance of the flow rate for a long enough period to overcome the inertia of the gauge used for its measurement.

Spirometry (Dynamic Lung Volumes)

Spirometry remains the single most useful lung function test in clinical practice. The patient breathes in as far as he can to total lung capacity, then breathes out to full expiration into a spirometer. The volume of gas exhaled is the vital capacity (VC). Usually the patient is asked to breathe out as hard and as fast as possible. During this forced expiration the volume of gas exhaled is recorded on a graph against time. This graph is the spirogram.

From the spirogram the following are routinely measured: forced expired volume in one second (FEV_1), forced vital capacity

(FVC). In airways obstruction, the ratio FEV_1/FVC is reduced below 75 per cent. A reduction in this ratio suggests obstruction in the large airways or severe disease of the small airways. When the obstruction is limited to the small airways, the disease must be extensive before it can be detected by this measurement.

A number of other measurements can also be made from the same graph although these are less valuable clinically. These are the maximum mid-expiratory flow rate (MEFR), which is the average rate of gas flow during the exhalation of the middle half of the vital capacity, and the flow rates at 50, 25, 20 and 10 per cent of the vital capacity. These measurements are usually made from a flow volume curve which is obtained automatically from an electrical signal generated by the spirometer and is displayed on an oscilloscope. The flow volume curve is a convenient way of replotting the spirogram, and it is important to realize that it is no newer or more complicated than that (Figure 7).

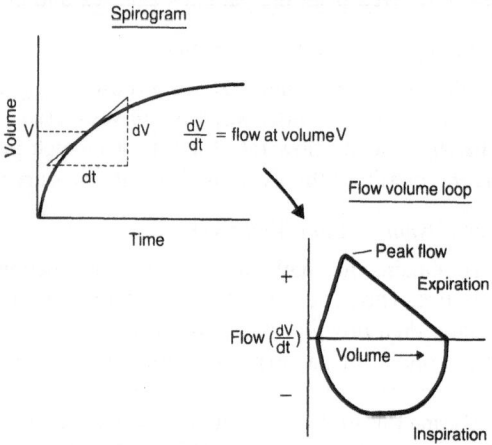

Figure 7. *The flow volume curve is another way of plotting the spirogram. Flow rates at each volume are calculated electronically by a circuit in the spirometer.*

The forced inspired volume in one second (FIV_1) can also be measured by asking the patient to take in a rapid deep breath from the moment the forced expiration is complete. Because the airways widen more on inspiration than expiration, inspiratory flow rates are higher than expiratory. The ratio FIV_1/FEV_1 is therefore greater than one. When this ratio is less than one it suggests extrathoracic airway obstruction, although muscular weakness and poor inspiratory effort can produce the same abnormality.

Static Lung Volumes

The total lung capacity (TLC), functional residual capacity (FRC) and residual volume (RV) are measured by body plethysmography or helium dilution (Webb 1980). The characteristic pattern in airways obstruction is an increase in the residual volume at the expense of vital capacity. This is due to early closure of the airways during expiration. The ratio of RV/TLC therefore rises. Lung volumes are helpful confirmatory evidence of airflow obstruction, but their measurement is not essential for diagnosis or for the assessment of the severity of the disease. They are particularly useful when two or more lung disorders coexist, e.g. chronic bronchitis and fibrosing alveolitis.

Gas Transfer

The diffusing capacity of the lung for carbon monoxide ($D_L$co) measures the amount of carbon monoxide transferred from the inspired gas to the blood during the test (usually 10 seconds breath holding). It is reduced in alveolar disease. Since most of the diseases of airflow obstruction spare the alveolus, the gas transfer is usually normal. In emphysema, the alveoli are dilated and destroyed and so the gas transfer is reduced. The test is therefore helpful in assessing the degree of emphysema in a patient with airflow obstruction. Unfortunately, gas mixing is poor in airway disease and this means that sometimes not all the carbon monoxide inhaled during the test reaches the alveoli. This can also reduce the gas transfer measured. The problem is avoided by correcting for the alveolar volume which is measured during the test. The corrected value is the gas transfer coefficient (Kco) which is a better estimate of the amount of emphysema.

Other Tests

Other tests may be used by specialist units to detect early airway abnormalities or to work out the functional disorder in detail in individual patients.

Compliance. This is measured by introducing a balloon into the oesophagus to estimate intrapleural pressure at different lung volumes. It may be done with the patient holding his breath (static compliance) or breathing normally (dynamic compliance). Increased compliance and a reduced maximum recoil pressure are seen in emphysema. The frequency dependence of compliance is claimed to be an indication of early small airway disease.

Closing volume, flow rates during helium breathing, single breath nitrogen washout. These tests have been developed to detect small airway disease early. They appear to do this, but are not yet being used routinely.

Blood Gases

Blood gas measurements are essential for the management of respiratory failure but have little place in routine management of the ambulant patient. They are discussed in Chapter 8.

Reversibility

Lung function tests are repeated after inhalation of 200 μg of salbutamol or an equivalent bronchodilator. An improvement in peak flow, FEV_1 or FVC is a measure of the reversibility of the airflow obstruction. Normals may improve 10 per cent and so an improvement of 15 per cent or more must be seen in order to diagnose asthma. Some reversibility is often observed in chronic bronchitis; this is seldom more than 10 per cent, but this may be very helpful to a patient incapacitated by breathlessness. Following bronchodilatation the TLC and RV may fall as the chest deflates.

Clinical Patterns

The diagnosis of each of the common diseases of airflow obstruction is made in a different way. Chronic bronchitis is defined in terms of clinical history, asthma by lung function, bronchiectasis is diagnosed by radiology and emphysema in terms of morbid anatomy. It is therefore not surprising that there is considerable overlap and these conditions often coexist. One way of getting round the problem is to lump all conditions except childhood asthma under a single diagnostic term. This is variously called chronic airways obstruction (COA) or chronic obstructive lung disease (COLD). By doing this, all precision is avoided and the diagnosis becomes almost meaningless. Worse, chronic obstructive lung disease implies that there actually is a single disease entity rather than the final common pathway resulting from a wide variety of conditions.

It is preferable to see the diseases of airflow obstruction as a spectrum (Figure 8). Within this spectrum, four well recognized

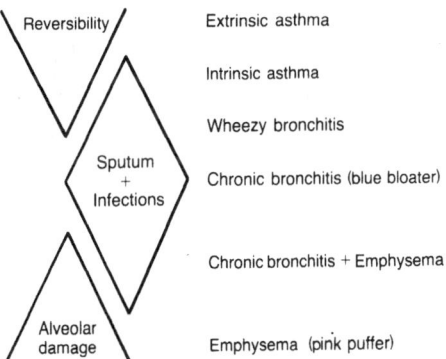

Figure 8. *The spectrum of airflow obstruction.*

clinical types are classically described. Although pure examples are seldom seen, they are useful as markers for position in the spectrum. These are the blue boater (Plate 1), the pink puffer, and the intrinsic and extrinsic asthmatic. The chief features of these types are listed in Table 1.

Table 1. Clinical archetypes in airflow obstruction.

(a) Reversible airflow obstruction

	Extrinsic asthma	Intrinsic asthma
Age (years)	<30	>30
Sex	M>F	F>M
Allergy	++	−
Infections	−	++
Nat. history	Improves	Worsens
Treatment	Bronchodilators	Steroids
Eosinophilia	Blood and sputum	Sputum only

(b) Irreversible airflow obstruction

	Blue bloater (Plate 1)	Pink puffer
	Chronic bronchitis	Emphysema
	P_{O_2} low	P_{O_2} maintained
	P_{CO_2} raised	P_{CO_2} low
	Cor pulmonale	No cor pulmonale
	Hypoventilation	Hyperventilation
	Overweight	Underweight
	Polycythaemia	No polycythaemia

3. Chronic Bronchitis

Definitions

Chronic bronchitis is usually defined as cough and sputum on most days for at least three months of the year in more than two successive years in the absence of any other cause (e.g. bronchiectasis). This definition is wide and does not imply infection or airflow obstruction. Three abnormalities occur in the disease:

1. Hypersecretion of mucus.
2. Infection resulting in purulent sputum.
3. Airflow obstruction.

A more precise diagnosis contains information about these abnormalities, e.g.:

Simple bronchitis—hypersecretion only.

Chronic mucopurulent bronchitis—hypersecretion with recurrent infections.

Chronic obstructive bronchitis—hypersecretion with airflow obstruction.

Occurrence

Chronic bronchitis is very common. It affects about one million people in the UK and causes about thirty thousand deaths a year. Mortality from the disease has been static for many years, but both the prevalence and the mortality are now beginning to fall.

Various factors are associated with an increased prevalence of the disease.

Nationality

Northern European countries, and the UK in particular, lead the world in chronic bronchitis. The reasons for this are not established but the following are important: air pollution, smoking habits and living conditions. Less important factors may be climate and an inherited predisposition to the disease.

Social Class

The prevalance of chronic bronchitis increases seven times from social class I to V, reflecting smoking habits, occupation and living conditions.

Town Versus Country

The prevalence of chronic bronchitis is lower in rural areas. This may be due to less frequent diagnosis as well as to cleaner air.

Causes

Smoking

Chronic bronchitis is very rare in non-smokers. The prevalence increases with the number of cigarettes smoked (Figure 9).

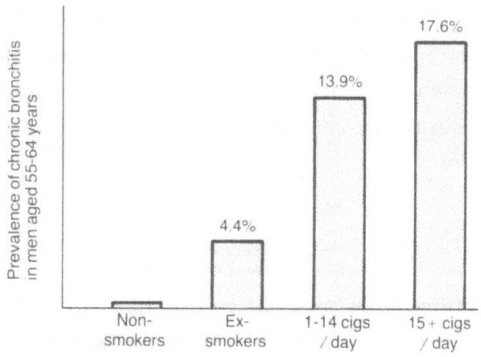

Figure 9. *The prevalence of chronic bronchitis in men aged 55 to 64 years (from Higgins, I. T. T.,* Br. Med. J., *1959,* **1**, *325).*

When smokers give up the habit, the prevalence of chronic bronchitis falls, as does mortality from the disease. Pipe and cigar smoking are probably safer, but this may be because less smoke is inhaled.

Atmospheric Pollution

There is a huge body of epidemiological evidence associating atmospheric pollution with the prevalence of and mortality from chronic bronchitis in the UK. The Clean Air Acts of 1956 and 1968 have considerably reduced pollution and this may be responsible for the decline in mortality from chronic bronchitis over the past few years.

Inherited Predisposition

Many smokers do not get chronic bronchitis. This may be partly due to differences in the way cigarettes are smoked, but it is possible that some smokers have an inherited predisposition.

Infection

Infection as a causative factor in chronic bronchitis is controversial. There is no doubt that severe childhood chest infections may cause later bronchiectasis, but an association between childhood infections and later chronic bronchitis is not universally accepted. Fletcher (1976) has established that, among chronic bronchitics, recurrent chest infections do not influence the severity or rate of progression of the airflow obstruction.

Pathology

Airways

Mucous gland hypertrophy (Plate 2). The mucous glands are in the submucosa of the larger airways. They normally make up less than 40 per cent of the total wall thickness, thus the gland : wall ratio (Reid index) is less than 0.4. In chronic bronchitis the Reid index increases and often exceeds 0.7 (Figure 10). Part of the excess mucus secretion comes from these hypertrophied glands.

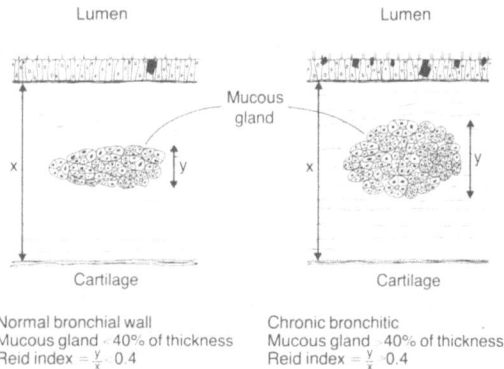

Figure 10. *The Reid index.*

Goblet Cell Metaplasia (Plate 3)

The normal bronchial mucosa is lined by ciliated columnar epithelium with an occasional mucus secreting goblet cell. The epithelial cells outnumber the goblet cells by 10:1 in the larger airways, and this ratio becomes 100:1 in the bronchioles. In chronic bronchitis there is probably an increase in the number of goblet cells in the peripheral airways.

Obliterative Bronchiolitis (Plate 4)

The small airways are narrowed with oedema and inflammatory cell infiltrate in the walls. Some of these airways become completely obliterated by inflammation, while others are occluded by mucus. The result is a reduction in the number of the small airways with narrowing of those that remain.

Alveoli

Since emphysema is associated with smoking, it is not surprising that many chronic bronchitics also have some degree of alveolar dilatation and destruction. However, this is very variable and the alveoli are often relatively normal.

Cardiovascular System

The heart and blood vessels show changes late in the disease. Muscular hypertrophy of the pulmonary arteries accompanies chronic pulmonary hypertension and the right ventricular wall becomes thicker. Some left ventricular hypertrophy is also common.

Pathophysiology

Airflow Obstruction

When airflow obstruction is present, it is due to narrowing of the large airways and narrowing and obliteration of the small airways. When emphysema coexists, then the reduced elastic recoil allows expiratory airway narrowing to occur earlier than normal, while the reduced alveolar pressure also contributes to the lower expiratory flow rates (see Chapter 1).

Gas Exchange

Gas exchange becomes abnormal in moderate and severe chronic obstructive bronchitis. The airways leading to some lung units are so narrowed that these alveoli are not well ventilated during tidal breathing. The result is a mismatching of ventilation and perfusion, with perfusion exceeding ventilation in some parts of the lung. This means that some blood passes through the lungs without coming into contact with enough air for gas exchange. In other words, there is an increase in the physiological shunt. This shunted blood tends to reduce the arterial P_{O_2} and increase the arterial P_{CO_2}. Both these changes stimulate the respiratory centre and ventilation increases. An increase in overall ventilation is efficient at blowing off CO_2 but has much less effect on O_2. As a result, the P_{O_2} remains low while the P_{CO_2} is normal or even a little below normal. When the disease is more advanced, ventilation is insufficient to blow off CO_2 and so the P_{CO_2} also rises (see Chapter 8). This is in part due to a reduction in central ventilatory drive.

The Work of Breathing

More muscular work is needed to overcome the airflow obstruction and also the respiratory muscles work inefficiently when the chest is overinflated. Eventually in severe disease, any increase in ventilation costs as much in oxygen consumption as it gains in better oxygenation.

Natural History

Hypersecretion

Many smokers never develop defined chronic bronchitis, but some increase in cough and sputum is almost invariable. The first event is a smoker's cough which may be noticed soon after starting smoking but more usually takes 10 or more years to develop. Some years after this, regular production of sputum begins, usually on rising in the morning. This hypersecretion helps colds to go down on to the chest, and the patient begins to have attacks of winter bronchitis. Eventually these lead to illnesses bad enough to keep the sufferer away from work and this is usually the first time he sees a doctor. If he continues smoking, the pattern continues with cough, sputum and recurrent infections, but not necessarily airflow obstruction or breathlessness. If he stops smoking, then cough and sputum production improve and often stop altogether. As the mucus hypersecretion lessens, chest infections become fewer.

Airflow Obstruction

The proportion of chronic bronchitics who also have airflow obstruction increases with age (Table 2). As the years pass, obstruction leads to breathlessness. About 50 per cent of patients with moderate breathlessness die within five years, while after the first episode of cor pulmonale, 67 per cent of patients die within

Table 2. The prevalence of airflow obstruction in chronic bronchitic males in a Colorado town (Mueller et al. 1971).

Age (years)	30–39	40–49	50–59	60–69	70+
$FEV_1/FVC < 60\%$ (%)	0	0	22	43	75

five years. Death is usually from cardiorespiratory failure complicating an acute infection; pulmonary emboli are a common contributory factor.

If the patient stops smoking, then the decline in lung function is much slower and is similar to the normal rate. However, he never recovers any of the previously lost lung function.

The natural history of chronic bronchitis is summarized in Figure 11.

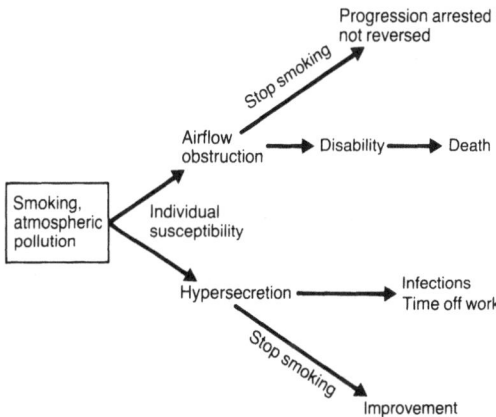

Figure 11. *The natural history of chronic bronchitis. (Modified from Fletcher et al.,* The Natural History of Chronic Bronchitis and Emphysema, *Oxford University Press, Oxford, 1976.)*

Complications

Acute Exacerbations

Episodes of acute purulent bronchitis become increasingly frequent as the disease progresses. Many episodes are triggered by a viral infection which damages the respiratory mucosa, and this allows a bacterial infection to become established. The pathogens

are almost invariably *Haemophilus influenzae* and *Strep.*
pneumoniae. These organisms are present as commensals in
mucopurulent sputum and become pathogenic during bouts of
acute bronchitis, although sometimes infection occurs with a new
strain.

During an exacerbation, airflow obstruction increases but lung
function usually returns to its previous level after recovery. In
patients whose lung function is already severely compromised
before the exacerbation, the increase in airflow obstruction may
cause respiratory failure, cor pulmonale or death. In this way,
influenza epidemics and periods of cold foggy weather are associated with dramatic rises in bronchitis mortality.

Pneumonia, lung abscess, empyema and tuberculosis occasionally complicate chronic bronchitis, but they are surprisingly rare.

Cor Pulmonale

Heart failure develops as a result of:

1. Pulmonary hypertension. Hypoxic pulmonary vasoconstriction
increases the pulmonary vascular resistance. Reduction in the
pulmonary vascular bed also plays a part when emphysema coexists.

2. Myocardial hypoxia, resulting in poor ventricular function.

3. Salt and water retention. CO_2 retention causes acidosis. The
extra hydrogen ions are excreted by the kidney in exchange for
sodium ions. Water is retained with the sodium.

Respiratory Failure

See Chapter 8.

Pneumothorax

Pneumothorax is not uncommon and can be life-threatening in a
patient with poor ventilatory function. Rupture of subpleural
blebs or bullae, which occur more commonly when emphysema is
present, is probably the cause.

Polycythaemia

Chronic severe hypoxia leads to an increased red cell mass in some patients. The haemoglobin may rise to higher than 20 g/dl and the haematocrit to over 60 per cent. Polycythaemia increases the oxygen carrying capacity of the blood and initially this may be beneficial, but eventually the increase in viscosity of the blood outweighs the benefit of the increase in its oxygen content.

Pulmonary Embolism

Pulmonary embolism is common in the terminal stages of the disease. Predisposing factors are cardiac failure, immobility and polycythaemia.

Peptic Ulcers

Peptic ulcers are common in chronic bronchitics. Possible factors associated with peptic ulcers are stress, smoking, oral cortico-steroids and hypoxia.

Clinical Features

Symptoms

Cough and Sputum

Most smokers consider cough and sputum as normal and do not count them as significant symptoms. Only when they change dramatically or become incapacitating will they bring a patient to see a doctor. The cough is most noticeable first thing in the morning, especially in the winter, but eventually is present throughout the day and may interfere with sleep. Exercise and change of posture may increase cough and expectoration.

Sputum is usually clear or white between attacks and becomes thicker and more colourful during infections. Typically, it becomes more copious and turns yellow, green or creamy. The patient is usually aware of any change. Occasionally the sputum is streaked with blood during an exacerbation. Frank haemoptysis suggests bronchial carcinoma or bronchiectasis.

Breathlessness

Initially the patient will only notice breathlessness during exacer-bations and on unusual exertion, but this worsens until he is breathless on walking on the flat and finally at rest. The complaint of breathlessness varies a great deal between different bronchitics and correlates poorly with lung function.

Infections

The patient usually complains of a cold which goes onto his chest. There is an increase in cough and the sputum becomes purulent. A fever and general malaise are usually, but by no means constantly, present. Breathlessness increases over the normal level but again this is variable, some patients may deteriorate into severe respiratory failure without noticing any increase in breathlessness.

Chest Pain

Transient chest pain is relatively common, and is usually due to a complication such as rib fracture, pleurisy, pulmonary infarction, tracheitis or pneumothorax. Persistent pain is not a feature of chronic bronchitis and another disorder such as bronchial carcinoma should be considered.

Physical Signs

Many chronic bronchitics have no abnormal physical signs. Abnormalities develop as airflow obstruction progresses. Airway disease causes wheezing, especially on expiration, and crackles, most marked in early inspiration. As a result of air trapping, the chest becomes hyperinflated with a hyper-resonant percussion note and the liver and cardiac dullness are lost. These are the only abnormalities in the majority of patients. When the obstruction is severe enough to cause respiratory failure, the low Po_2, and sometimes high Pco_2, affect the cardiovascular and central nervous systems, producing cyanosis, peripheral vasodilatation, right ventricular failure, confusion and asterixis (see Chapter 8).

Investigations

Radiology

The chest radiograph is usually normal. Abnormalities when present are due to complications. Pneumonic shadowing may be

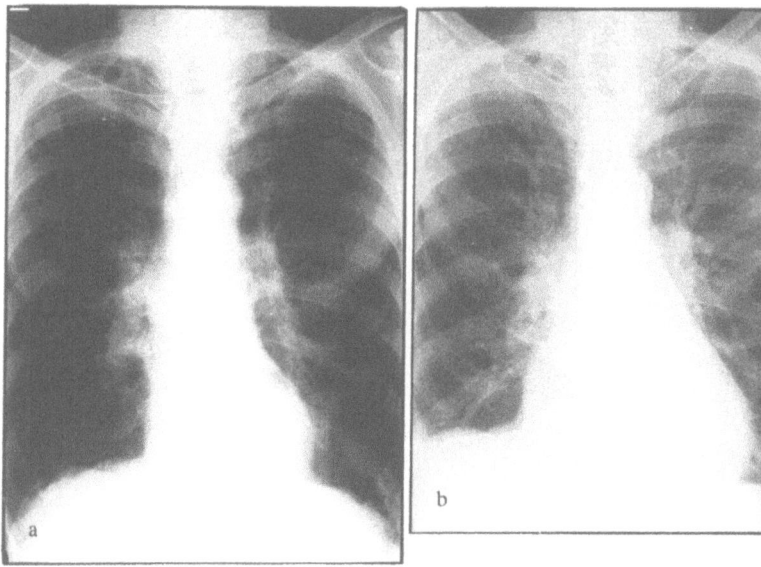

Figure 12. *(a) Chest radiograph in chronic bronchitis. (b) Chest radiograph of the same patient after the development of cor pulmonale.*

seen during an acute exacerbation; cardiomegaly or pulmonary venous congestion indicate cor pulmonale (Figure 12). When emphysema coexists, the diaphragms are low and flat (Figure 13), the heart shadow is long and thin, and the lung markings are diminished.

Haematology

The haemoglobin and haemotocrit are raised in secondary polycythaemia, but this is relatively rare. The white count may rise transiently during infections but is usually normal. An eosinophilia suggests an asthmatic component to the disease. The ESR may rise following infections and is low in cor pulmonale.

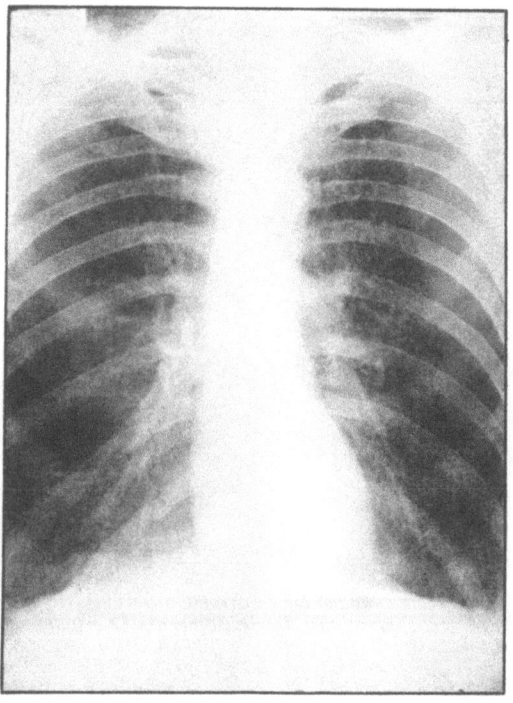

Figure 13. *Chest radiograph in emphysema. Note the low flat diaphragms, vertical heart and poor peripheral markings, especially in the right midzone.*

Biochemistry

Biochemical investigations seldom contribute much to the management of chronic bronchitis. A raised urea is usually due to diuretic therapy. A low serum potassium may be caused by diuretics or steroids. When recurrent infections are a problem, it is worth checking the immunoglobulin levels.

Bacteriology and Serology

Sputum microscopy can be useful as sputum purulence is occasionally due to eosinophils, which suggest an asthmatic component.

H. influenzae and *S. pneumoniae* are by far the commonest bacterial pathogens cultured from infected sputum, but in many patients with an acute exacerbation, no organism can be isolated.

Lung Function Tests

Functional Abnormality

The typical pattern of abnormality is a reduction in FEV_1 and FVC with a FEV_1/FVC ratio less than 75 per cent. The TLC is normal or high, and the RV is high producing a raised RV/TLC ratio. The gas transfer is normal, but low when there is significant emphysema. The peak flow rate is low. During exacerbations, the lung function tests deteriorate, but otherwise there is little variability and the improvement following inhaled bronchodilator is less than 10 per cent. A greater change than this indicates asthma.

Full lung function testing is helpful in defining functional impairment and assessing the degree of reversibility of airflow obstruction. This should be done when the patient first notices breathlessness. Thereafter, it is helpful to monitor the progression of the disease and for this, spirometry alone is adequate. Regular peak flow readings are an alternative, being easier to perform, but give less information.

Exercise Tolerance

A patient's assessment of his disability is imprecise. The McGavin 12-minute walking test gives a much better objective measurement. In this, the patient walks up and down a corridor at his own pace, stopping if necessary. The total distance covered in 12 minutes is measured. The distance is very repeatable, and gives a good assessment of the patient's disability. It can be used to assess the effect of treatment and has an advantage over spirometry in that it measures what the treatment is intended to do, namely to improve the chronic bronchitic's mobility.

Treatment

Treatment can be considered in two ways. The prevention of progression of disease in those who are only mildly affected and the relief of symptoms in those with severe disease. Unfortunately, once severe airflow obstruction has developed, treatment will have very little effect on mortality.

Prevention of Progression

Progression can be prevented by breathing clean air and stopping smoking. Environmental pollution has been considerably reduced by the Clean Air Acts of 1956 and 1968 and working conditions are also improving, but these advances have not been matched by changes in smoking habits. If a patient with chronic obstructive bronchitis stops smoking, the rate of deterioration of his lung function will be halved.

Prevention of infective exacerbations probably has little effect on disease progression, but may reduce the amount of time off work. Influenza vaccination should be recommended in October or November.

Symptomatic Treatment

Cough and Sputum

Inhalations, expectorants and cough suppressants are often ridiculed as there is little scientific basis for their use. However, patients usually find they are helpful, and most of these preparations are cheap.

Breathlessness

Bronchodilators and steroids. Some improvement in airflow obstruction can usually be achieved with drugs. Ideally, the effect of β adrenergic stimulants, parasympathetic blocking drugs and steroids should be assessed, and then treatment continued with the effective agent. Symptomatic improvement is unreliable, especially with steroids which may improve general wellbeing, and so some measurement of lung function must be made. Spirometry is sufficient for this. The assessment is best done when the patient first complains of breathlessness.

Patients with moderate or severe breathlessness should have a trial of prednisone, 30 mg daily for two weeks, and spirometry should then be repeated. If there is a greater than five per cent increase in FEV_1 or FVC *and* symptomatic improvement, long-term steroid therapy should be considered. Beclomethasone, two puffs q.d.s., will usually maintain the spirometric improvement, and only if this fails should oral prednisone be continued.

Oxygen. Home oxygen can help the severely breathless patient, and a small refillable portable supply can improve his mobility. Continuous oxygen therapy may also help cor pulmonale.

Acute Exacerbations

Antibiotics should be taken as soon as the sputum changes. It is best for the patient to have a supply of antibiotics at home and so avoid delay. Tetracycline 250 mg q.d.s., ampicillin 500 mg q.d.s., amoxycillin 250 mg t.d.s., or cotrimoxazole, two tablets b.d., are equally effective. There are theoretical reasons for preferring erythromycin 250 mg q.d.s., since this will also be effective against mycoplasma and the rare staphylococcal infection. The antibiotics should be continued for 10 days.

Hospital admission is not usually necessary, but should be considered if physiotherapy is required to bring up sputum. Confusion, disorientation or drowsiness all suggest respiratory failure and hospital admission is then urgent.

Cor Pulmonale

Ankle swelling alone may need no treatment, but if troublesome, usually responds to a thiazide diuretic such as bendrofluazide 5 to 10 mg daily with potassium supplements. Frusemide 40 to 120 mg daily and spironolactone 100 to 200 mg daily are needed in resistant cases. There is often an element of left ventricular failure as well and breathlessness may improve with adequate diuresis. Digoxin is probably of little benefit unless uncontrolled atrial fibrillation coexists. Digoxin can be dangerous during an exacerbation when hypoxia, acidosis and hypokalaemia all sensitize the myocardium to arrhythmias.

Long-term controlled oxygen for 12 to 15 hours daily has been shown to reduce pulmonary artery pressure. This may improve cor pulmonale and therefore mortality. Until long-term benefits have been assessed, this treatment should not be recommended as it is inconvenient and expensive.

Polycythaemia

When the haematocrit exceeds 60 per cent, the patient may benefit from venesection. One or two pints are removed over an hour and replaced with Dextran 40. When successful, the patient notices improved exercise tolerance and mental function.

Respiratory Failure

See Chapter 8.

4. Emphysema and Bullae

Emphysema

Definition

Emphysema is an increase in size of the air spaces distal to the terminal bronchiole with destruction of their walls. Since emphysema is defined, on morbid anatomy, a specimen of lung tissue must be examined before the diagnosis can be made with certainty.

Classification can be confusing since many of the morbid anatomical patterns described have little to do with clinical disease. From the clinical point of view, only two forms of emphysema are important.

Centriacinar

The destruction is confined to the centre of an acinus while the more peripheral parts are normal. The respiratory bronchiole and its immediately surrounding alveoli are enlarged. This is particularly associated with chronic bronchitis and pneumoconiosis. A mild degree of centriacinar emphysema may be found in lungs of normal individuals dying of unrelated causes, and it increases with age.

Panacinar (Plate 5)

The destruction of alveolar walls occurs throughout the acinus and is not related to the feeding airway. This can be an advanced form of centriacinar emphysema associated with chronic bronchitis, but sometimes occurs in isolation as 'primary' emphysema. The best example of this is in α_1 antitrypsin deficiency.

Centriacinar emphysema usually starts in the upper parts of the lung, while panacinar emphysema is predominantly basal.

Causes

Emphysema probably occurs because the balance between tissue breakdown and repair is disturbed. There are three important factors in this process.

1. Local release of tissue damaging enzymes from macrophages and white cells.

2. Circulating inhibitors of these enzymes, e.g. α_1 antitrypsin.

3. The structure of lung collagen. Abnormal collagen biochemistry in some patients with 'primary' emphysema has been reported, but this needs confirmation.

Pathophysiology

Airflow Obstruction

The widespread loss of alveolar walls reduces their elastic recoil. The alveolar pressure is reduced as well as the radial traction in the airway walls. The result of this is a considerable reduction in expiratory flow rates. Airways close early in expiration with air trapping. During inspiration, the airways open to a nearly normal size and so inspiratory flow rates are relatively normal. Because some airways are closed or narrow throughout tidal breathing, the alveoli they supply may receive little air. These alveoli are ventilated via the pores of Kohn which connect them to adjacent alveoli. This is called collateral air drift.

Gas Exchange

The pulmonary capillary bed is reduced and so the surface area available for gas exchange is less than normal. As a result, some of the inspired air may reach the periphery of the lung, but may fail to make full contact with capillary blood. The ventilation may then exceed perfusion in parts of the lung and this mismatching has the effect of increasing the physiological dead space.

The blood passing through the lungs moves faster in emphysema than normally since there are so few capillaries to accommodate the cardiac output. Therefore blood is in contact with alveolar gas for a shorter time than normal and complete equilibration may not occur. This leads to a fall in Po_2 on exercise when the cardiac output rises.

Abnormalities of arterial blood gases in emphysema differ from those in chronic bronchitis. The Po_2 is usually above 60 mm Hg and the Pco_2 low. This is partly because of the differences in gas exchange.

Cardiac Output

Cardiac output tends to fall as the pulmonary capillary bed is attenuated. However, since the Po_2 is well maintained, hypoxic vasoconstriction does not occur and pulmonary hypertension and cor pulmonale are unusual.

Compliance

Loss of alveolar walls makes the lungs more compliant. As a result they expand more under the influence of a negative intrathoracic pressure. Total lung capacity is therefore increased and the chest is overinflated.

Work of Breathing

The work of breathing increases because of the increase in expiratory airways resistance and the mechanical disadvantage suffered by the respiratory muscles working on a hyperinflated chest.

Clinical Features

Symptoms

Cough and sputum. These are often present, especially during exacerbations. However, many patients are not chronic sputum producers and therefore do not have chronic bronchitis.

Breathlessness. This is usually the dominant symptom. Patients with severe airflow obstruction may be unable to do more than walk across the room, while many chronic bronchitics with the same FEV_1 can get out and lead a relatively normal life.

Weight loss. This is common and may precede gross breathlessness. Poor appetite, difficulty in eating because of breathlessness and increased work of breathing are possible explanations.

Physical Signs

The chest is hyperinflated and breathlessness is obvious, with use of accessory muscles of respiration and gasping for air. The percussion note is hyper-resonant with loss of cardiac and liver dullness. Expiration is prolonged during tidal breathing and the breath sounds are quiet. Expiratory wheezing and fine early inspiratory crackles may be heard but these are inconstant. Because of the increase in air between the heart and the chest wall, the heart sounds are louder in the epigastrium than over the praecordium.

Investigations

Radiology (see Figure 13)

The essential abnormalities are overinflation with diminished vascular markings. Overinflation is judged on low flat diaphragms with a thin vertical heart and an enlarged retrosternal space on the lateral film.

Lung Function Tests

Expiratory flow rates (FEV_1, peak flow, FEV_1/FVC) are reduced and the RV/TLC ratio increased as in all forms of airflow obstruction. Abnormalities which particularly suggest emphysema are:

1. Raised TLC.

2. Low CO diffusion factor ($D_L co$) and CO diffusion coefficient (Kco).

3. High compliance.

The most valuable of these is the Kco since it is easy to measure and correlates best with the amount of emphysema.

Treatment

This is essentially the same as for chronic bronchitis (see Chapter

3). There is seldom any significant response to corticosteroids, although β stimulants often produce a little improvement in FVC with symptomatic benefit. Breathlessness is the most disabling symptom and some relief of this can be attempted as follows:

Oxygen

A home supply of oxygen will improve mobility and can be used to relieve symptoms. A small portable cylinder which can be refilled can improve a patient's mobility outside the home.

Walking Aids

Frames with wheels have been designed to take part of the patient's weight while walking, but these are only useful on a smooth surface. An electrically powered wheelchair can transform a patient's life, but unfortunately few can afford them.

α_1 Antitrypsin Deficiency

α_1 antitrypsin deficiency is a rare inherited abnormality. α_1 antitrypsin is a protein, formed in the liver, which is normally released into the blood and acts as an inhibitor of a wide range of proteolytic enzymes. The inheritance is basically a mendelian dominant with many co-dominant alleles. Each allele has been given a letter according to the electrophoretic mobility of the protein and the phenotype of an individual is expressed as two of these letters. The common alleles are M, S and Z and the common phenotypes MM (86 per cent of a caucasian population), MS (nine per cent), and MZ (three per cent). The phenotype MM has normal levels of α_1 antitrypsin, while ZZ has very low levels. MS, SS and MZ are intermediate.

About one in 5000 individuals is ZZ and tends to have liver disease in childhood or emphysema in adult life.

α_1 Antitrypsin Deficient Emphysema

Patients present with severe panacinar emphysema in their 30s or 40s and die from respiratory failure within the next few years. The emphysema is predominantly basal and smoking appears to speed up its development. It is likely that the α_1 antitrypsin deficiency allows increased protein breakdown within the lungs and is not simply a genetic marker of disease. About one to three per cent of patients with emphysema have α_1 antitrypsin deficiency. The diagnosis is made by demonstrating a low serum α_1 antitrypsin level and confirmed by phenotyping.

Management

The patient's relatives should be seen and serum specimens taken for phenotyping. Any individual with a ZZ phenotype is likely to develop emphysema. Smoking should therefore be forbidden. All children of a ZZ will carry the Z allelle and if such an individual marries an MZ heterozygote, half their offspring will be at serious risk. Genetic counselling is important since ZZ homozygotes are usually of reproductive age. The management of the emphysema itself is conducted along conventional lines.

Heterozygotes

The phenotypes MS, MZ have intermediate levels of α_1 antitrypsin. Detailed studies of such individuals have shown a slight impairment of lung function, especially among smokers. It is possible that they have an increased risk of developing chronic bronchitis or emphysema.

Bullae (Plate 6)

Definition

A bulla is an airspace greater than one centimetre in diameter within the lung. Smaller airspaces are called blebs and the division is arbitrary.

Pathology

Bullae are found in association with emphysema, chronic bronchitis and pulmonary fibrosis. Since the air inside the bulla is not resorbed, there is always a connection between the bulla and the bronchial tree.

Pathogenesis

Emphysema

A small airspace is formed by the destruction of alveolar walls. Air continues to enter the space by collateral drift but does not leave during expiration because of airways closure. As the space enlarges, the surface tension of its wall decreases, predisposing to further enlargement.

Valve Mechanism

An airway may be distorted or narrowed by disease and so allow air to enter the bulla more easily than it leaves. The distortion may be caused by fibrosis or another bulla. Endobronchial sarcoidosis rarely acts as a valve.

Traction

In lung fibrosis, parts of the lung may shrink relative to others. This traction leads to bullae formation in the more normal lung. Coexisting distortion of airways may contribute.

Pathophysiology

The bulla occupies space and distorts surrounding lung.

Airflow Obstruction

Airflow obstruction is often present as part of the underlying disease (emphysema, chronic bronchitis). In addition, a major airway may be distorted and narrowed by the bulla.

Gas Exchange

There is negligible ventilation or perfusion within a bulla and so it does not contribute to gas exchange. However, surrounding alveoli may be compressed and their ventilation impaired. As a result, the total alveolar surface available for gas exchange is reduced. Ventilation and perfusion are likely to be poorly matched around the bulla.

Complications

Pneumothorax is particularly likely to occur with subpleural bullae. Infection is rare, but when present a fluid level can be seen in the bulla. Following infection, the bulla sometimes disappears, presumably because the connections with bronchial tree are obliterated.

Clinical Features

Bullae are usually asymptomatic but may contribute to the breathlessness caused by the underlying disease. Chest pain has been occasionally attributed to a bulla.

Signs are those of the underlying disease.

Investigations

Radiology and Lung Scans

The diagnosis is made on the PA and lateral chest radiographs (Figure 14). The bullae are better delineated by whole lung tomography or bronchography although the latter is seldom needed.

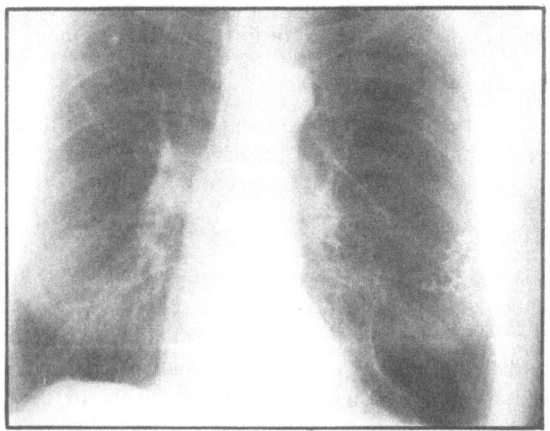

Figure 14. *Chest radiograph of a patient with multiple bullae.*

Ventilation and perfusion scans can help to delineate the bullae but add little to tomography.

Lung Function Tests

These measure the function of the non-bullous lung and indicate the severity of the underlying disorder. Regional studies using mass spectrometry and fibreoptic bronchoscopy are elegant and give further detail of the function of individual lobes or segments. Unfortunately, no test yet can make the required measurement, namely what would be the function of the surrounding lung if the bulla were removed.

Treatment

Treatment is only required if the patient is breathless. The aim is to obliterate the bullae and so improve the function of the surrounding lung. This can be done surgically by plication or resection. Some patients are dramatically improved but many are not, and with an operative mortality of around 10 per cent, the decision whether or not to operate is very difficult.

5. Bronchiectasis and Cystic Fibrosis

Bronchiectasis

Definition

Bronchiectasis means dilated bronchi, which may be demonstrated by bronchograms or morbid anatomical examination. The term does not imply any symptoms of disease.

Pathology (Plate 7)

The bronchi are dilated because of damage to their walls and there is usually evidence of chronic inflammation. The essential changes are destruction of normal tissues with fibrous replacement and variable inflammatory cell infiltrate. This is seen in all layers of the bronchial wall and it extends peribronchially. The bronchial arteries enlarge in bronchiectasis and become tortuous. Anastomoses with the pulmonary circulation are increased.

Pathogenesis

The bronchial wall is damaged by inflammation. This can be due to specific infections, e.g. pertussis, measles, tuberculosis, but non-specific infections which persist or recur are the commoner cause. This may happen for several reasons.

Bronchial Obstruction

Foreign bodies, bronchial adenomas and pressure from enlarged lymph nodes cause collapse of the distal lung with recurrent infections. This results in local bronchiectasis.

Abnormal Mucociliary Clearance

Cystic fibrosis and ciliary abnormalities may lead to generalized bronchiectasis. Abnormal cilia have been demonstrated in Kartagener's syndrome.

Immune Deficiency

Identifiable deficiency states are rare but malnutrition and poor living conditions produce relative immuno-incompetence. This may account in part for bronchiectasis following whooping cough and measles pneumonia in childhood, which now occurs less commonly.

Complications

Infections

Acute exacerbations with increase in cough, sputum and sputum purulence occur as in chronic bronchitis. The pulmonary parenchyma is often involved producing pneumonia and pleurisy. Occasionally the infection spreads to the pleural space as an empyema. The commonest organisms are *Haemophilus influenzae* and *Strep. pneumonia*, but staphylococci, *Klebsiella* and *Pseudomonas* are not unusual. Sinusitis commonly accompanies bronchiectasis and may be due to a defect in handling respiratory tract infections at all sites because of poor local defences.

Haemoptysis

Small volumes of blood in the sputum are common and unimportant. Occasionally profuse haemoptysis is life-threatening, due to either alveolar flooding or exsanguination. The source is usually a hypertrophied bronchial artery.

Brain Abscess, Amyloidosis

Since the advent of antibiotics these complications seldom occur.

Clinical Features

Symptoms

Cough and sputum, often first noted in childhood, are the hallmarks of bronchiectasis and usually persist throughout the year. The sputum is usually purulent and becomes thicker and green or yellow during infective exacerbations. Occasionally it clears completely following antibiotics but it returns within a few weeks. Upper lobe bronchiectasis, especially secondary to old tuberculosis, may not be associated with cough and sputum, presumably because gravity keeps the bronchi well drained. The sputum is often blood-stained, especially during an infective episode. Massive bleeding is rare. Haemoptysis may be the presenting symptom of bronchiectasis. Widespread bronchiectasis eventually causes breathlessness but most bronchiectatics lead a normal active life. Attacks of wheezy breathlessness with bronchiectasis suggests bronchopulmonary aspergillosis.

Signs

Clubbing is common; in particular it accompanies widespread

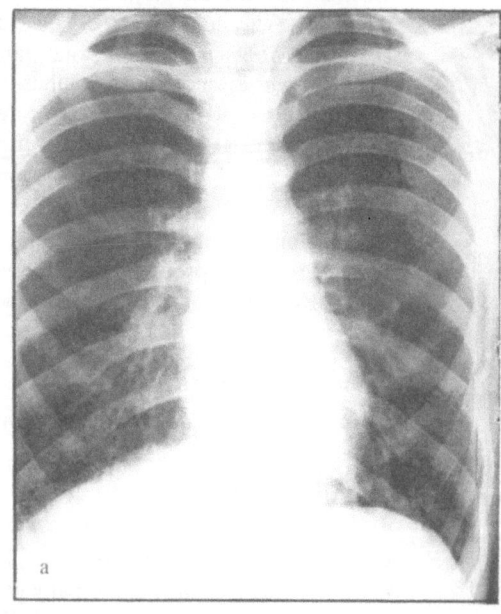

Figure 15. *(a) Chest radiograph of a patient with left lower lobe bronchiectasis. (b) Magnified view of the left lower lobe showing parallel line shadows. (c) Bronchogram from the same patient confirming the bronchiectasis.*

bronchiectasis with bronchial artery hypertrophy. Moist mid-inspiratory crackles are heard over the affected lung. They are often accompanied by short high-pitched wheezes.

Investigations

Radiology

PA and lateral chest radiographs are abnormal in over 90 per cent of patients with bronchiectasis (Figure 15). Bronchial wall thickening produces tramline shadows especially in the lower zones. Peripheral ring shadows are formed by cystic bronchi. Patchy peripheral shadowing is caused by pneumonia, collapse or fibrosis.

Bronchograms make the definitive diagnosis, but they are not usually necessary unless surgery is contemplated, when they are

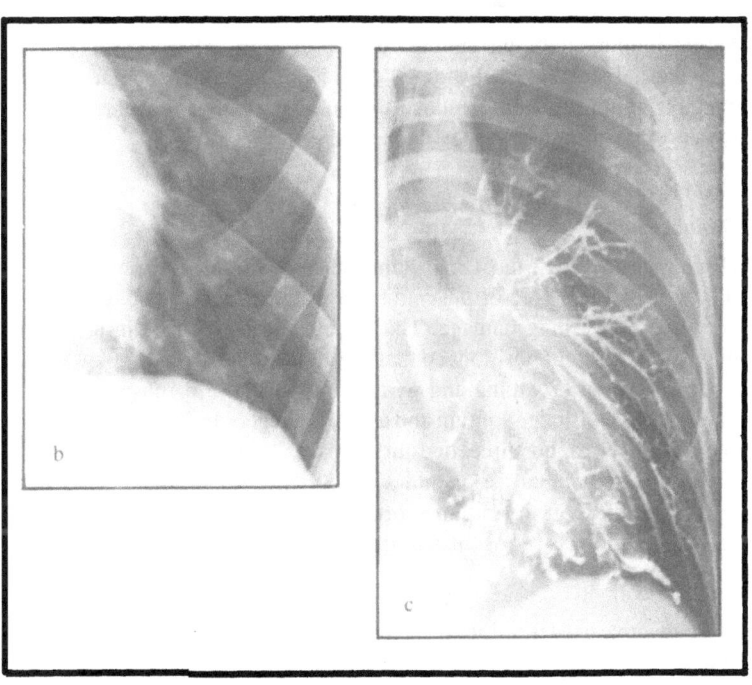

used to define the extent of the disease. Bronchiectasis affecting the proximal bronchi with a normal peripheral pattern suggests bronchopulmonary aspergillosis. When bronchiectasis is diagnosed, the sinuses should be radiographed.

Lung Function Tests

Airflow obstruction is usual and causes a low FEV_1, FEV_1/FVC and peak flow. When there is extensive collapse and fibrosis, the TLC and vital capacity are also reduced. The RV is usually high as a result of the airflow obstruction. The D_Lco is often low and reflects the amount of lung damage. In aspergillosis the obstruction is partially reversible.

Lung function tests are of most value in assessing a patient's respiratory reserve if surgery is considered.

Immune Deficiency

Serum immunoglobulins should be measured in patients with bronchiectasis. Occasionally low levels are found and then regular gammaglobulin injections reduce the number of infections and may prevent progressive lung damage.

Treatment

Drainage

Drainage is the single most important measure. The aim is to keep the bronchial tree free of pus and so prevent infective episodes and progressive lung damage. The patient is taught to lie in a number of different positions so that the affected lobes can drain. Coughing, deep breathing and percussion by spouse or physiotherapist help dislodge sputum and assist drainage. Ideally, drainage should be done three or four times daily, but it is time-consuming and embarrassing and a compromise is often necessary. When little or no sputum is produced, the patient can stop drainage, but must restart at the first sign of an infection.

Antibiotics

Most infective exacerbations respond to tetracycline or ampicillin and these may be started without sputum culture results. The

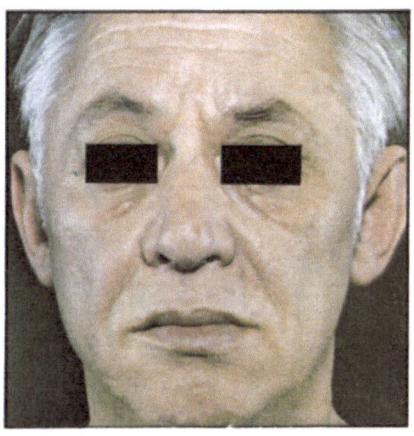

Plate 1. *A blue bloater. (Courtesy of Dr F. H. Scadding, Middlesex Hospital, London.)*

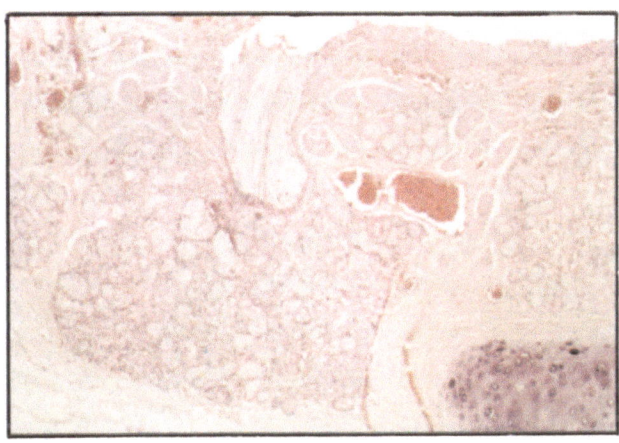

Plate 2. *Histology of the bronchus in chronic bronchitis, demonstrating mucous gland hypertrophy. (Courtesy of Dr B. Heard, Brompton Hospital, London.)*

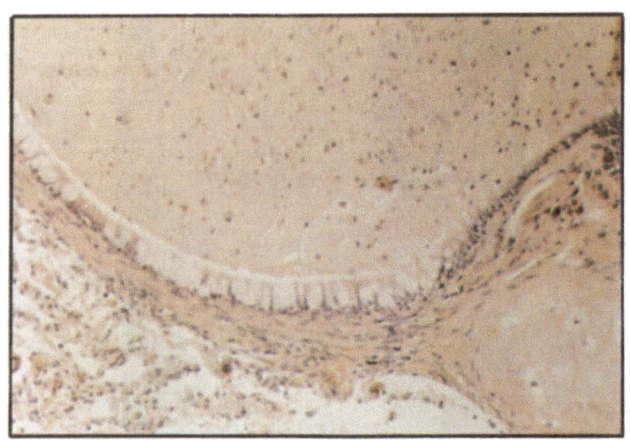

Plate 3. *Goblet cell metaplasia in chronic bronchitis. (Courtesy of Dr B. Heard, Brompton Hospital, London.)*

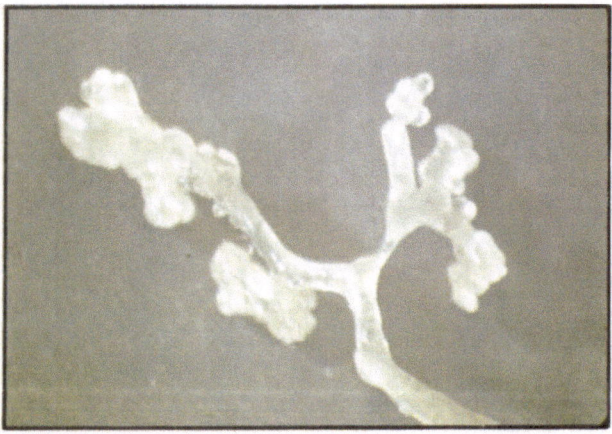

Plate 4. *Airway obliteration and narrowing in chronic bronchitis. (Courtesy of Dr B. Heard, Brompton Hospital, London.)*

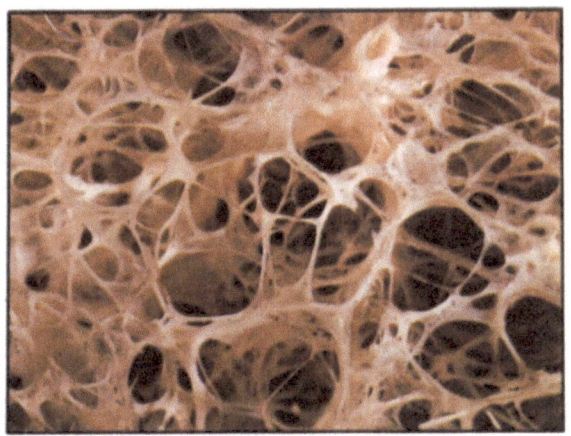

Plate 5. *Low power magnification of emphysematous lung. (Courtesy of Dr B. Heard, Brompton Hospital, London.)*

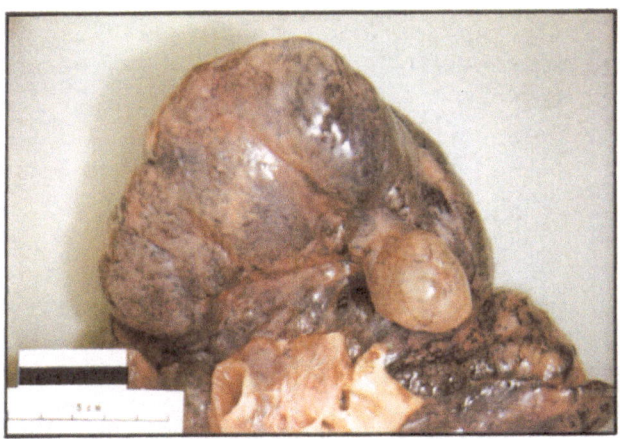

Plate 6. *Operation specimen showing multiple bullae. (Courtesy of Dr B. Heard, Brompton Hospital, London.)*

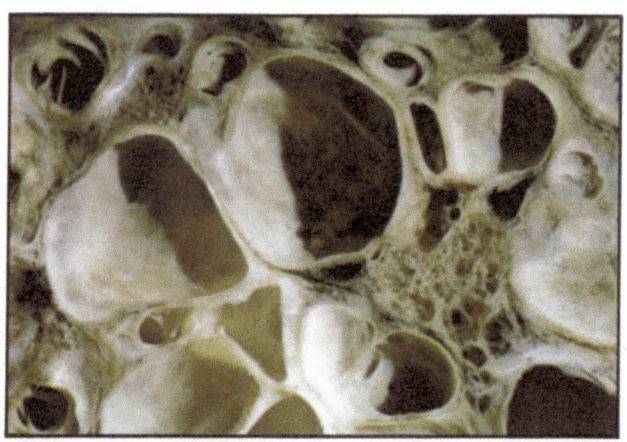

Plate 7. *Widely dilated airways in bronchiectasis. (Courtesy of Dr B. Heard, Brompton Hospital, London.)*

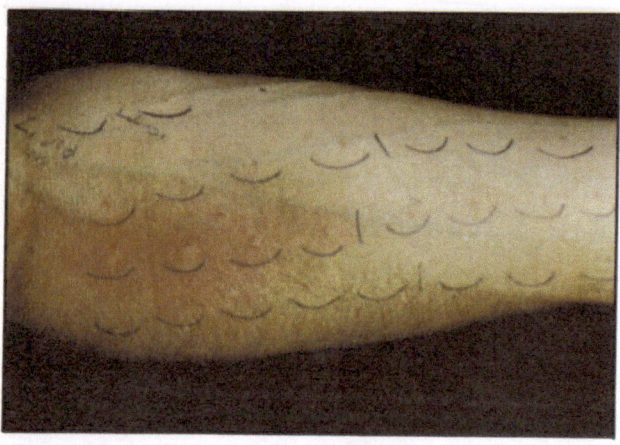

Plate 8. *Positive prick tests showing typical wheal and flare. (Courtesy of Dr Sherwood Burge, Brompton Hospital, London.)*

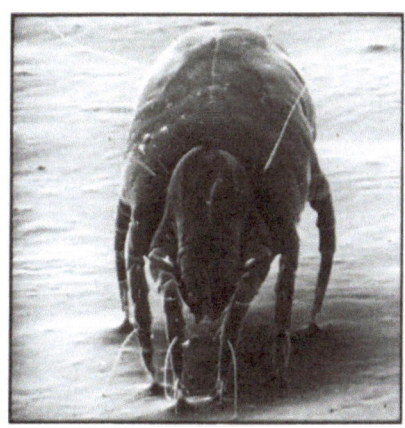

Plate 9. *House dust mite,* Dermatophagoides pteronyssinus *(Crown copyright, Ministry of Agriculture Pest Infestation Control Laboratories. Kindly supplied by Ms V. Cowper.)*

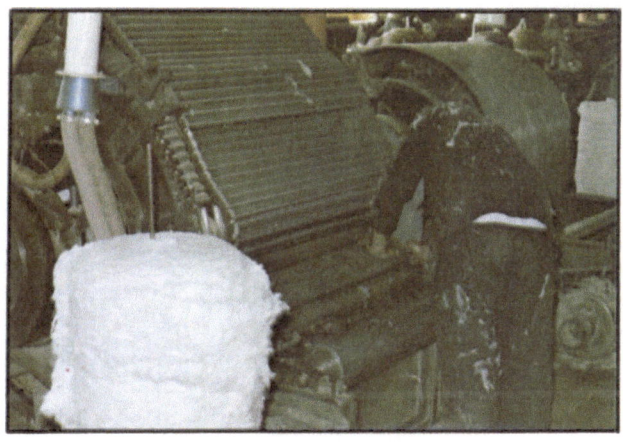

Plate 10. *Cotton carding in a factory. (Courtesy of Dr Sherwood Burge, Brompton Hospital, London.)*

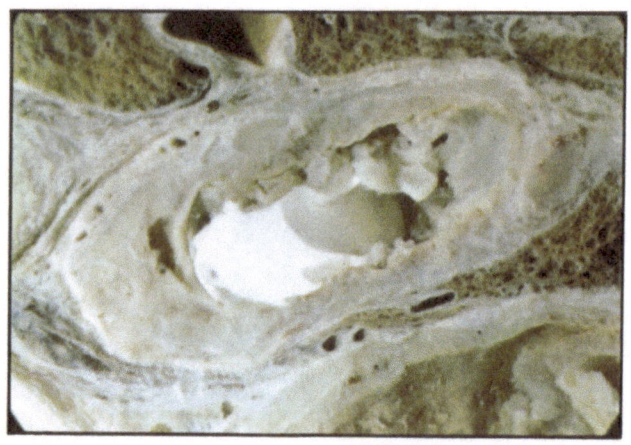

Plate 11. *Thickened airway wall in asthma. (Courtesy of Dr B. Heard, Brompton Hospital, London.)*

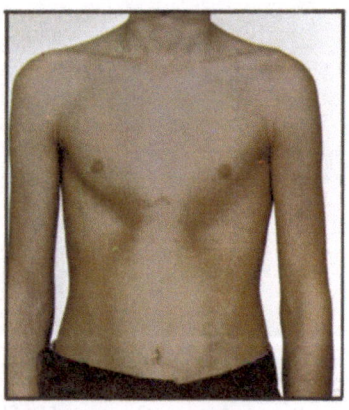

Plate 12. *Rib deformity (pigeon chest) in chronic asthma.*

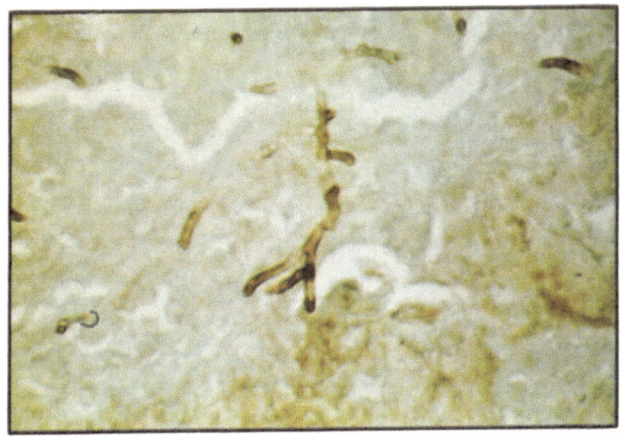

Plate 13. *Hyphae of* Aspergillus fumigatus *in sputum plug from patient with allergic bronchopulmonary aspergillosis. (Courtesy of Dr Newman Taylor, Brompton Hospital, London.)*

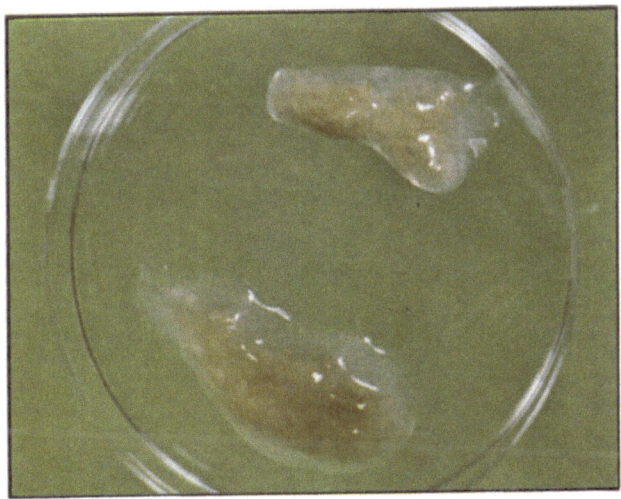

Plate 14. Aspergillus *sputum plug. (Courtesy of Dr Newman Taylor, Brompton Hospital, London.)*

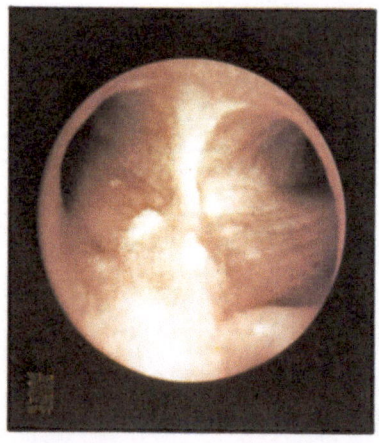

Plate 15. *Endobronchial sarcoidosis: note subcarinal node enlargement and the white plaques. (Courtesy of Dr P. Stradling, Hammersmith Hospital, London.)*

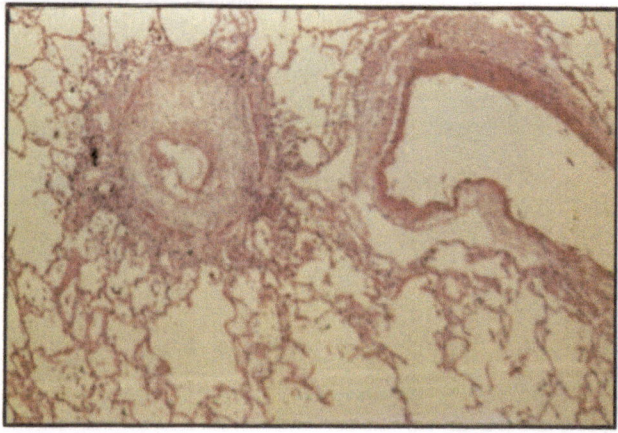

Plate 16. *Bronchiolitis showing narrowing and inflammation of a small airway.*

patient should keep a supply of antibiotics at home and start a course as soon as the infection begins. If the infection does not respond, sputum should be cultured and further antibiotics directed at the organisms grown. Occasionally an exacerbation persists and then admission to hospital for physiotherapy and more intensive antibiotics is helpful. Long-term maintenance antibiotics are seldom worthwhile.

Surgery

Surgery is only valuable for localized bronchiectasis in a patient with adequate lung function. The affected lobe or segment is removed and all symptoms cease. Lobectomy or bronchial artery ligation is occasionally necessary for massive haemoptysis.

Cystic Fibrosis

Definition

An inherited disorder of exocrine gland secretion resulting in:

1. High sweat sodium and chloride.
2. Chronic bronchopulmonary sepsis.
3. Pancreatic insufficiency.

Genetics

Transmission is by a recessive gene. The homozygote has the disease, while the heterozygote is entirely healthy. The gene is carried by about one in 25 caucasians and about one in 2000 live births is a homozygote with the disease. Cystic fibrosis is therefore the commonest inherited disease among Europeans. The basic biochemical defect is unknown and at present there is no reliable way of identifying heterozygotes.

Pathology

Sputum accumulates in the bronchi. This is mucoid initially but eventually becomes infected. In early life, *Staph. aureus* is the commonest pathogen but this is replaced by *Haemophilus influenzae* or *Pseudomonas* as the child gets older. This leads to damage of the bronchial walls and bronchiectasis. Many of the smaller airways are blocked or obliterated. All segments of the lung are involved but in contrast to other forms of bronchiectasis, the upper zones are the worst affected and in early disease may be the only site of bronchiectasis. Pneumonia, lung abscess and empyema all occur but are surprisingly rare; the alveoli are relatively normal. Chronic sinus infection and nasal polyps are common.

Complications

Infective exacerbations are signalled by increase in cough and sputum, usually with fever, systemic upset and a decline in lung function.

Pneumothorax is rare in childhood, but becomes more common in adolescent and adult life, affecting about 30 per cent of patients.

Haemoptysis is common, blood-streaked sputum being reported in over 70 per cent of adolescent patients. Severe life-threatening haemoptysis occurs in under five per cent of patients, but may be the terminal event.

Eventually most patients die in *respiratory failure* in the course of an infective exacerbation. Chronic hypercapnic respiratory failure occurs but is rare. Once the full clinical picture of respiratory failure develops the prognosis is very bad and aggressive treatment is seldom justified.

Ten per cent of patients present in infancy with intestinal obstruction from the viscid meconium (*meconium ileus*). A similar event occurs occasionally in childhood and adolescence when impaction of inspissated faeces produces obstruction.

Malabsorption is usually controlled by pancreatic enzyme replacement, but most patients are underweight.

Diabetes develops in about 20 per cent of older patients. This is controlled by standard measures. Ketoacidosis is not a problem.

Cirrhosis and portal hypertension occur in fewer than 10 per cent of patients.

The high sweat sodium levels can lead to *heat stroke*, but this can be prevented by salt supplements.

Clinical Features

In childhood meconium ileus, diarrhoea, recurrent bronchitis or failure to thrive are the presenting symptoms. Pancreatic supplements control the malabsorption and the chief symptoms are then cough and sputum with infective exacerbations. Breathlessness becomes common in adolescence. Chest pain is due to musculoskeletal injury from coughing or pneumothorax. Pleurisy complicating infections is rare.

There may be no abnormal physical signs. As the airways become progressively damaged, so the non-specific signs of airflow obstruction develop: hyperinflation, hyper-resonant percussion note, prolonged expiration and wheezing. The earliest abnormality is fine crackles in the first half of inspiration, chiefly in the upper zones. Finger clubbing is nearly always present. The sputum is strikingly thicker and more tenacious than in other chest diseases, the colour varies from grey to brown or green.

The abdomen is usually normal but distension, hepatosplenomegaly or signs of obstruction may be found.

Investigations

Radiology

The chest radiograph is normal in early life but becomes progressively abnormal as the lungs are damaged. Parallel line shadows representing thickened bronchial walls appear in the upper zones (Figure 16). These are joined by ring shadows and small patchy opacities until eventually all the lung fields are diffusely abnormal.

Bronchograms are not necessary and since they may make drainage of secretions more difficult they should not be performed.

Haematology

The haemoglobin is normal although the serum iron is usually low. The white count may rise during infections but is otherwise normal.

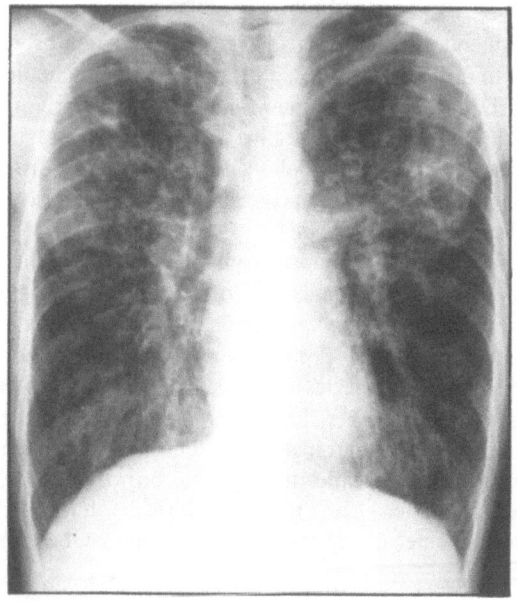

Figure 16. *Chest radiograph in cystic fibrosis showing the widespread shadowing most marked in the upper zones.*

Biochemistry

The sweat sodium level is high. In children a level over 70 mmol/l is diagnostic. In adults the level must be over 90 mmol/l on three occasions. In doubtful cases, fludrocortisone 4 mg daily is given for five days and the test repeated; in cystic fibrosis the sweat sodium level does not fall.

Bacteriology

Sputum culture is the most important investigation once the diagnosis is made. The same organism is usually grown from a patient over a long period. *Staph. aureus, Haemophilus* and *Pseudomonas* are the commonest pathogens but *Proteus* and anaerobes occasionally give problems. Tuberculosis is very rare.

Lung Function Tests

The functional pattern is similar to that of bronchiectasis. Spirometry should be done frequently to assess progress and prognosis. A sharp decline in spirometric volumes is by itself an indication for intensive treatment.

Treatment

Drainage

Drainage is essential, and the patient and his relatives must be taught the techniques by a physiotherapist. Physiotherapy is then carried out for as long or as often as necessary to keep the bronchi clear of retained secretions. This may be only once daily but often has to be done as often as three or four times daily, each session lasting about half an hour. More physiotherapy is needed during infections. Regular energetic sports are an effective and enjoyable form of physiotherapy and should be encouraged whenever possible.

Antibiotics

Maintenance antibiotics are often given but the evidence that these help is still lacking. The choice of these antibiotics is relatively simple when *Staph. aureus* or *Haemophilus* is grown, as oral cloxacillin or ampicillin can be taken regularly. It is wise not to give tetracycline to children, to avoid discoloration of teeth.

Bronchodilators

β stimulants improve the airflow obstruction and may aid mucociliary clearance. These should be given regularly if there is objective benefit. Steroids are seldom helpful.

Supplements

Pancreatic enzyme supplements are essential and the correct dose is that which abolishes diarrhoea and allows weight gain. Regular fat soluble vitamin supplements should be taken.

Complications

Pneumothorax. A small pneumothorax usually resolves without treatment. Otherwise intercostal drainage is necessary. If a pneumothorax recurs, it is likely to continue recurring and surgical pleurodesis or pleurectomy should be performed if lung function allows.

Haemoptysis. Massive or continuous bleeding is rare but life-threatening. Bronchial artery embolization or ligation must be considered.

Meconium ileus. Surgery is usually necessary in infancy. The older patient with intestinal obstruction commonly improves with rehydration and administration of acetyl cysteine or gastrografin.

General Management

Most patients can attend normal schools and obtain normal employment. However, many will die before 20 years of age and most before 40 years, and this inevitably causes many social and psychological problems. The medical social worker and careers officer are an essential part of the team necessary to help these patients get the most out of their short and difficult lives.

6. Asthma and Pulmonary Eosinophilia

Asthma

Definition

Asthma is variable airflow obstruction. Some authorities insist on 20 per cent variability, while others are content with 10 per cent. Fifteen per cent is a reasonable compromise, but it is best not to be dogmatic as there is considerable overlap in respiratory diseases (see Chapter 2).

Prevalence

Asthma is common throughout the world, affecting up to five per cent of children. In childhood it is twice as common in boys as in girls, but in middle life this is reversed, with women outnumbering men by two to one or more. The first symptom usually occurs in childhood, although a quarter of women asthmatics have their first attack in middle age.

Causes and Pathogenesis

Asthmatic airflow obstruction can be seen as a simple chain of cause and effect. An environmental trigger factor acts on a susceptible individual. A series of immunological or neurological events takes place which produces chemical mediators. These mediators act on smooth muscle and airway narrowing results.

This simple scheme is probably true for all forms of asthma, although the actual triggers and mediators may differ. In allergic asthma, the details have been well worked out, while in late onset 'intrinsic' asthma, the trigger factors, host factors and mediators are largely unknown.

Trigger Factors

Allergy. This is an immunological hyper-reactivity to an antigen. Type I allergy is associated with high circulating levels of IgE and, after sensitization to an antigen, specific IgE is found bound to mast cells. On challenge with the antigen, the mast cell degranulates and releases mediators. Type I allergy is demonstrated by positive prick tests (Plate 8) and the relevance of a particular allergen to asthma can be confirmed by inhalational challenge testing; asthma develops within 15 minutes of challenge. This is the commonest trigger in childhood. The allergens are different in different countries, but in temperate climates house dust, the house dust mite (*Dermatophagoides pteronyssinus*) (Plate 9), pollens and moulds (especially *Aspergillus fumigatus*) are the most important. Animal proteins are important in households with pets.

Type III hypersensitivity involves the formation of immune complexes when the antigen combines with precipitating antibody. If these complexes remain in the tissues, they provoke inflammation and tissue damage. When this occurs in the bronchial walls, the airways become narrowed and asthma develops. The commonest antigen to do this is *Aspergillus fumigatus*. Type III allergy is demonstrated by a six to eight hour (Arthus) reaction to an intradermal injection of antigen and its relevance to asthma confirmed by inhalational challenge testing; asthma develops six to eight hours after challenge. Precipitating antibodies are found in the serum.

Infection. Respiratory tract infections are usually due to viruses. When these involve the lower respiratory tract they provoke asthma in susceptible subjects. Sometimes the first bout of asthma follows an infection, and thereafter the patient develops wheezing in response to many different triggers.

Exercise. In normals exercise causes slight sustained bronchodilatation. By way of contrast, in some asthmatics asthma develops five to fifteen minutes after the start of exercise. This particularly affects young atopic subjects. Recent work has suggested that inspiration of cold air may be the main cause of exercise-induced asthma.

Irritants, chemicals and cold. Mediator release and the autonomic nervous system can both be implicated. Irritants cause cough and asthma very rapidly after inhalation and it is likely that these effects are mediated by the parasympathetic nervous system. Atropine can often block this response. Many chemicals and allergens used in industry also cause asthma, e.g. colophony resin in solder flux, byssinosis caused by cotton bracts (Plate 10) and toluene di-isocyanates in paint manufacture. Cold may provoke a mixed response in that atropine may block the asthma, but some patients also develop urticaria on exposure of the skin to cold and this suggests local mediator release.

Psychological factors. While these are undoubtedly important in a few patients, the factors discussed above usually dominate.

Host Factors

Atopy. The tendency to develop type I allergic reactions is called atopy. Atopic individuals have an increased prevalence of asthma, eczema, urticaria and hay fever. However, atopy is much more common than the diseases it causes. About 25 per cent of normal individuals have one or more positive skin prick tests and this contrasts with a prevalence of asthma of less than five per cent. There is often a strong history of atopic disease in the family of an asthmatic. Atopy may develop as a result of antigen exposure in infancy and breast feeding seems to reduce the incidence of atopic disease in later life.

Bronchial hyper-reactivity. A wide variety of inflammatory mediators, such as histamine and prostaglandins, produce bronchoconstriction when they are inhaled. This affects both asthmatics and normal individuals, but at very different doses. A normal subject may have to inhale 1000 times more histamine than an asthmatic to produce the same effect. Bronchial hyper-reactivity is a prominent feature in asthma and is relatively non-specific since it happens in response to a wide range of insults including irritants and cold.

Menstruation and menopause. Asthma is often worse premenstrually and at the menopause. Conversely, it may improve during pregnancy. Steroid hormone changes may be involved, although this is not proved.

Heredity. Undoubtedly asthma runs in families as does atopy. The mode of inheritance of these traits suggests that many genes are involved with variable expression.

Mediators

When mast cells degranulate a large number of vasoactive amines and lipids are released: histamine, slow reacting substance of anaphylaxis, prostaglandins and thromboxanes, 5 HT, bradykinin and eosinophil chemotactic factor (ECFA). The picture is confused since some of these substances cause bronchodilatation, e.g. PGE_1, while others cause bronchoconstriction, e.g. $PGF_{2\alpha}$. The net effect of these mediators is to cause bronchoconstriction, and in some instances the nervous system is involved.

Airway Narrowing

The bronchial smooth muscle contracts when the intracellular level of cyclic AMP falls and relaxes when the level rises. It is probable that the intracellular level of cyclic GMP has the opposite effect. The mediators released from mast cells act on the smooth muscle by altering the intracellular level of cyclic AMP and probably GMP. The mediators also change the cyclic nucleotide levels in mast cells, an increase in cyclic AMP depressing mediator release. The overall effect is to cause bronchoconstriction as well as feeding back on the mast cells to inhibit further mediator release. The same changes are brought about by an increase in parasympathetic nervous tone.

The changes also affect pulmonary blood vessels with contraction of smooth muscle and increase in capillary permeability. This results in mucosal oedema which narrows the airway. Mucus secretion increases and some small airways become blocked. Airflow is thus further impaired.

Pathology (Figure 17 and Plate 11)

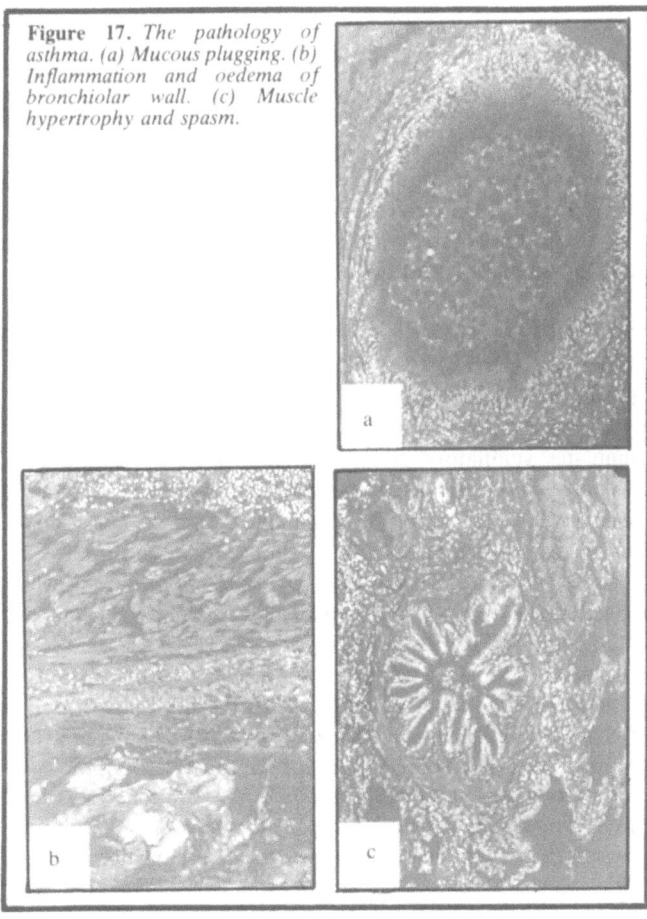

Figure 17. *The pathology of asthma. (a) Mucous plugging. (b) Inflammation and oedema of bronchiolar wall. (c) Muscle hypertrophy and spasm.*

The bronchial mucosa is infiltrated with eosinophils and the bronchial smooth muscle is hypertrophied. There is a variable increase in the number of goblet cells and the bronchial mucous glands may be hypertrophied, although this may be a reflection of chronic bronchitis which often coexists in the middle-aged asthmatic. There is excess mucus in the airways, and when death has been caused by a prolonged bout of asthma many airways are blocked by mucous plugs. The alveoli are normal.

Pathophysiology

Airflow Obstruction

Diffuse airway narrowing reduces expiratory flow rates. When many airways are plugged by mucus, this contributes to the reduction. The narrowed airways close early in expiration and the residual volume is therefore increased.

Gas Exchange

There is mismatching of ventilation and perfusion. Many alveoli receive little ventilation in relation to their perfusion and so the physiological shunt increases. As a result the Po_2 is low. This stimulates ventilatory drive, ventilation increases and CO_2 is blown off. The Pco_2 is usually low. When the overall ventilation is insufficient, less CO_2 is blown off and the Pco_2 rises. This is due to the severity of the airflow obstruction combined with muscular weakness. Muscular weakness becomes important during a prolonged attack due to exhaustion, acidosis and the inefficiency of acting on a hyperinflated chest.

When asthma is treated with bronchodilators, smooth muscle relaxes in blood vessels as well as airways. This has two separate effects on gas exchange. First, the ventilation of alveoli increases and thus ventilation perfusion ratios improve. Second, the vasodilatation cancels the effects of hypoxic vasoconstriction and more blood flows to relatively hypoxic alveoli. As a result, the physiological shunt may actually increase although ventilation perfusion ratios improve. This is shown by a fall in Po_2 following bronchodilator therapy.

Work of Breathing

During an attack the work of breathing may increase tenfold, partly because of the airflow obstruction and partly because of the mechanical disadvantage of the respiratory muscles.

Cardiovascular System

The pulmonary artery pressure may increase acutely during a bout of asthma due to hypoxic vasoconstriction; increased intrathoracic pressure may play a part. An electrocardiogram taken during an attack may show P pulmonale and right axis deviation which revert to normal after treatment. Cor pulmonale is very rare in asthma and when it occurs there is usually coexisting irreversible airflow obstruction from chronic bronchitis.

Natural History

Onset and Resolution

Asthma usually starts in childhood. Onset before the age of 12 years is common and thereafter it becomes progressively less frequent. Patients continue to present sporadically with their first symptoms in their 20s and 30s but this is rare. The incidence then rises again in middle life, especially in women. After the age of 60, a new diagnosis of asthma is again unusual but sporadic cases continue to occur into old age.

Children with asthma usually improve during their teens and many patients will be free of symptoms by the age of 20 years. A few unfortunate asthmatics continue to have symptoms intermittently throughout life. The patients who lose their asthma by the age of 20 often remain free of the disease indefinitely. However, a few will have a recurrence of asthma in later life, usually around 40 to 50, and when it returns it tends to persist. Similarly, asthma presenting for the first time in middle life tends to persist and to become progressively more severe.

Patterns of Asthma

Labile asthma. Some labile asthmatics show an entirely chaotic pattern, but more usually there is a regular diurnal change with the lowest peak flows being recorded early in the morning. These morning dips tend to be exaggerated when patients are recovering from a bout of asthma and may be related to asthma deaths. Patients in hospital dying of asthma usually do so during the early hours of the morning a few days after their admission when they appear to be improving. The reason for these morning dips is not known but circadian changes in neuroendocrine functions may play a part. Normal individuals show similar, but much smaller, diurnal changes in peak flow. Asthma deaths outside hospital also occur in labile asthmatics who may be entirely well 30 minutes before the fatal attack. Labile asthmatics are often young and atopic; they respond dramatically to inhaled β stimulants, and their asthma may be chiefly mediated by bronchial muscle contraction.

Drifting asthma. This is the usual pattern in late onset asthmatics. A deterioration is followed by slow improvement. These patients respond less dramatically to bronchodilators and are less often atopic than the labile asthmatics. It is possible that their asthma is mediated by mucosal oedema and secretions more than by bronchial muscle contraction.

Complications

Infections

Acute bronchitis and pneumonia may precipitate or complicate an attack of asthma. Mucous plugging and poor clearance of secretions from narrowed airways predispose to infection and the common respiratory pathogens *Streptococcus pneumoniae* and *Haemophilus influenzae* are usually involved.

Pneumothorax and Pneumomediastinum

Both pneumothorax and pneumomediastinum are infrequent complications, presumably due to rupture of a subpleural bleb secondary to changes in intrathoracic pressure caused by the asthma.

Segmental Collapse

Occasionally mucous plugging of a large airway produces segmental or lobar collapse which results in increased breathlessness. Diagnosis is difficult without a chest radiograph. Re-expansion usually follows physiotherapy and bronchodilator therapy, but bronchoscopy and suction may be needed.

Chest Deformity and Stunting (Plate 12)

Chest deformity and stunting are now rare. In the past children with long-standing uncontrolled asthma developed pigeon chests, and stunting was due to excess oral corticosteroids.

Clinical Features (Table 3)

Table 3. Clinical indices of severe asthma.

Heart rate	>110/min
Blood pressure paradox	>20 mm Hg
Peak flow	<100 l/min
Talking	Sentences short or unfinished
P_{O_2}	<55 mm Hg

Symptoms

Breathlessness. Episodes of wheezy breathlessness brought on by some trigger are typical. Often no trigger factor can be identified. The patient may describe asthma as tightness in the chest rather than breathlessness. This is usually worst on rising in the morning and may wake the patient in the early hours. Descriptions vary so much that no particular pattern of symptoms is needed for the diagnosis and the episodic nature may not be obvious at all.

The complaint of breathlessness is not a good index of severity. Some patients with severe obstruction become accustomed to it and do not mention breathlessness at all.

Cough. The triggers which provoke asthma often provoke cough as well, and in some patients this is the dominant symptom. The cough is usually episodic and unproductive. Cough is such a common symptom in adults that underlying asthma may well pass unrecognized. A persistent troublesome cough in a child should raise the possibility of asthma and should be investigated.

Sputum. Most asthmatics have no sputum except in the course of respiratory tract infections. However, middle-aged asthmatics may produce sputum persistently between bouts and the distinction between asthma and chronic bronchitis becomes blurred. During an attack, purulent sputum usually represents an infection, although occasionally all the cells are eosinophils, in which case the purulence is purely allergic. Occasionally plugs of sputum, which may represent bronchial casts, are coughed up. This is particularly a feature of bronchopulmonary aspergillosis. A few patients cough large quantities of watery sputum for some time after a bout of asthma. The cause of this bronchorrhoea is unknown but it may respond to a course of oral steroids.

Physical Signs

Wheeze and breathlessness. Continuous musical noises can be heard at the mouth and through the chest wall. They occur diffusely throughout the chest, chiefly during expiration which is prolonged. When an asthmatic is well, there is usually no wheeze, although it may be brought out by asking the patient to breathe deeply and rapidly. Wheezing is not a good index of severity of asthma since a certain minimum airflow is needed to make the noise. When an attack is so severe that there is negligible airflow, the chest may become silent.

Breathlessness causes an increased respiratory rate with increased respiratory effort. A fair measure of the severity of a bout of asthma is the extent to which the breathlessness interferes with talking. When only short sentences are possible, the attack is severe. At worst, talking becomes monosyllabic.

Hyperinflation. This is gross in young asthmatics during an attack. The middle-aged asthmatic may show little hyperinflation, even when the attack is severe.

Tachycardia. This is present during an attack and is a good measure of its severity. Unfortunately, drugs complicate this sign. Nevertheless, a heart rate of over 110/min suggests a severe attack. In children, rates of 130 to 150/min are not unusual.

Peak flow rate. This should be a routine part of the physical examination in asthma. A peak flow of under 100 l/min indicates severe asthma. In dangerous attacks, the peak flow is usually unrecordable.

Blood pressure. The difference between the systolic blood pressure in expiration and inspiration is called the amount of paradox; this is a reflection of the intrathoracic pressure changes during respiration. In normals, there is 5 to 10 mm Hg of paradox while in asthma this increases to 15 to 40 mm Hg and is a measure of pressures needed to generate airflow. It is therefore a good index of the severity of asthma unless the patient becomes exhausted.

Investigations

Radiology (Figure 18)

The only consistent radiographic abnormality is hyperinflation during bouts of asthma. The diaphragms are low but well rounded and the pulmonary vasculature normal. A radiograph should always be taken in a severe or prolonged attack of asthma to exclude complications (pneumonia, pneumothorax, atelectasis).

Lung Function Tests

The diagnosis is confirmed by demonstrating more than 15 per cent improvement in PEFR, FEV_1 or FVC following bronchodilator therapy (10 to 15 min after inhaled β stimulant or after two to three weeks of oral corticosteroids). Other lung function tests are not essential.

Immunology

Skin prick tests. These establish the atopic status of the individual. A positive prick test does not prove that asthma is caused by the

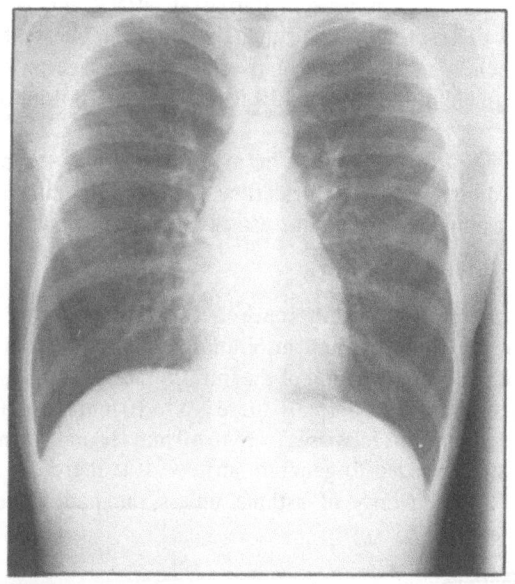

Figure 18. *Chest radiograph in asthma showing hyperinflation with rounded diaphragm and normal vascular markings.*

allergen, although it is likely. A drop of solution of allergen is placed on the forearm and pricked into the epidermis with a sharp needle. A 3 mm wheal represents a positive reaction. There is a large number of allergens available for testing but few are needed for general use. In the UK house dust, house dust mite, grass pollen and *Aspergillus fumigatus* are adequate.

Inhalation challenge testing. This establishes the relevance of an individual allergen to a patient's asthma. This is only rarely necessary, e.g. for industrial asthma induced by a single chemical encountered only at work, and should be done by specialist units.

Precipitating antibodies to Aspergillus. See page 73.

Haematology

An eosinophilia suggests allergic asthma although other causes, e.g. drugs and intestinal parasites, should also be considered. An eosinophilia with chest radiograph shadowing is usually due to aspergillosis (see page 72). The ESR is often high following infection but persistent elevation raises the possibility of polyarteritis nodosa.

Treatment

Recommended regimens are shown in Table 4.

Table 4. Recommended regimens.

Allergic		
Occasional	*Frequent*	*Frequent and Severe*
Inhaled bronchodilator, 2 puffs p.r.n.	Sodium cromoglycate (Intal) caps. q.d.s.	Sodium cromoglycate (Intal) caps. ⎫
	Inhaled bronchodilator, 2 puffs p.r.n.–q.d.s.	Inhaled bronchodilator, 2 puffs ⎬ q.d.s.
		Inhaled beclomethasone, 2 puffs ⎭
		Rarely—oral steroids

Non-allergic		
Mild	*Moderate*	*Severe*
Inhaled bronchodilator, 2 puffs p.r.n.–q.d.s.	Inhaled bronchodilator, 2 puffs q.d.s.	As moderate +
	Inhaled beclomethasone, 2 puffs q.d.s.	Prednisone 5 to 15 mg alt. days

Prevention

Avoid triggers. Exposure to allergens can be minimized especially when one is known to be dominant. House dust can be reduced by damp dusting, vacuum cleaning, and by using linoleum flooring and plastic furniture coverings instead of carpet and upholstery. Mattresses and pillows should be made of synthetic materials or alternatively enclosed in polythene covers. When a prick test is positive for cat, dog or some other household pet, it is worth trying to establish that the pet actually provokes asthma before recommending its removal.

Sodium cromoglycate (Intal). This compound prevents asthma triggered by allergen exposure and exercise. It is seldom effective against other triggers, although cold and irritants are unpredictable. In vitro, the drug prevents the degranulation of sensitized mast cells on exposure to allergen and it probably works by limiting mediator release. Therefore it must be taken before allergen exposure, and it has no effect on an established attack of asthma. There is no effective oral preparation and so the drug has to be inhaled as a fine dust from a Spinhaler. Children under the age of six years often find this difficult.

Sodium cromoglycate is prescribed as one capsule inhaled three or four times daily for allergic asthma or one capsule five to 10 minutes before exercise for exercise-induced asthma. Its effect continues for four to six hours. The chief disadvantage of the drug is that it must be taken regularly even when the patient has no asthma. In occasional patients, it actually provokes a bout of asthma, but otherwise is free of side effects. There is no convincing evidence that it helps middle-aged patients with non-allergic asthma even in high dosage.

Hyposensitization. There is no good evidence that hyposensitization works, except in the rare patient with asthma triggered by a single allergen, for example grass pollen.

Bronchodilators

β *stimulants*. Selective β_2 stimulants (salbutamol, terbutaline, rimiterol) have less effect on the heart than non-selective β stimulants (isoprenaline, orciprenaline, ephedrine) and the same effect on the bronchi and so should be preferred. There is very little difference between the different β_2 stimulants and the choice is made essentially on a cost and patient preference basis. There are, however, important differences in the formulations.

1. Inhalers put the drug where it is needed with little systemic absorption. The bronchodilatation is the same as by any other route but the systemic side effects are fewer. Maximum effect is achieved quickly (five to 15 minutes after inhalation) and lasts three to six hours, depending upon the drug. Difficulties arise when a patient does not use the inhaler efficiently and when asthma is so severe that airflow is insufficient to carry the drug into the lungs. All patients must be taught how to use the inhaler.

A fine tremor of the hands occasionally occurs but otherwise side effects are negligible. It is possible that cardiac arrhythmias were provoked by massive overuse of non-selective β stimulants in the past and that the freon propellant of the aerosol played some part in this. In practice, this overuse of the inhaler is not a problem with selective β_2 stimulants.

One to two puffs of the inhaler are taken either when needed or four times daily. When eight to 12 puffs are taken in one day, and the asthma remains poorly controlled, then other therapy is required.

2. Oral preparations have no pharmacological advantage over inhalers and are more likely to cause tremor and tachycardia. They should be used when the patient cannot use inhalers or finds them too inconvenient to take regularly. There is no purpose in giving tablets at the same time as an inhaler since either alone produces maximum bronchodilatation. The only exception to this is a long-acting tablet, e.g. salbutamol spandet, which can be taken at bedtime to provide bronchodilatation throughout the night.

3. Intravenous preparations are only necessary for severe attacks (see status asthmaticus, page 67).

Anticholinergic drugs. Atropine methonitrate and the related compound ipratropium bromide produce bronchodilatation similar to β stimulants in both amount and duration. Anticholinergic side effects prevent these drugs being used systemically but they can be taken by inhaler in the same way as β stimulants. They can be tried as additional treatment when other measures are inadequate.

Xanthines. These are local irritants and cannot be inhaled. Their main use is for acute severe attacks rather than in maintenance therapy. Aminophylline 250 mg IV can be given slowly as initial treatment for a severe asthma attack and may need to be continued as an infusion over the next 12 to 24 hours (see status asthmaticus, page 67). Aminophylline suppositories can be helpful in the same way, but their continued use may cause rectal irritation and proctitis. Xanthine drugs can cause nausea and cardiac arrhythmias.

Others. α blockers and E prostaglandins have theoretical appeal but no place in routine management. Antihistamines have no effect. Occasionally aspirin is an effective treatment, presumably acting by blocking the synthesis of prostaglandin $F_{2\alpha}$. Patients have often discovered the value of aspirin themselves and can be encouraged to go on using it. Unfortunately, in a few patients aspirin is a potent trigger producing severe and occasionally fatal asthma.

Steroids

Steroids are an extremely effective treatment although their mode of action is unknown. They are used in two ways: maintenance therapy and short courses for severe attacks.

Maintenance therapy is needed when asthma cannot be controlled by the measures described. Inhaled beclomethasone is taken one to two puffs four times daily regularly. Inhaled steroids are hardly absorbed and so the risk of long-term side effects is negligible. The only problems are poor inhaler technique and oropharyngeal candidiasis. This latter is troublesome in about 5 per cent of patients and can be abolished by amphotericin lozenges.

A few patients remain uncontrolled with inhaled steroids and need oral prednisolone 5 to 20 mg daily. These patients suffer from long-term steroid side effects and the benefit of the treatment must be balanced against this risk. The lowest maintenance dose possible is found by trial and error and most patients become adept at varying the dose according to their symptoms. Alternate day dosage is usually effective and reduces side effects. Regular inhaled beclomethasone probably helps keep the total oral steroid dose low. Drugs used for their steroid sparing effects in other diseases (e.g. azathioprine) have not been shown to do this in asthma. ACTH is only indicated for growing children whose asthma is uncontrolled by beclomethasone, since stunting of growth can be caused by prednisolone.

Short courses are necessary for any severe or prolonged attack. When the attack is especially severe, intravenous hydrocortisone is used (see status asthmaticus, page 67), otherwise oral prednisone is adequate. A reducing course, starting at 40 mg daily and reducing by 5 mg each day, is easy for the patient to remember, although occasionally it is necessary to maintain the high dose for a week or two before reducing. Patients already taking oral steroids do the same except that they reduce the dose to their normal maintenance level.

Hypnosis

This is very effective in some patients. It should be considered when asthma is particularly labile, when psychological factors appear important, when an attack is accompanied by more than usual anxiety and in any patient whose asthma is refractory to routine treatment.

Status Asthmaticus

Definition

Any attack of asthma which remains severe after initial treatment. This encompasses a child whose allergen-induced attack does not improve within an hour of inhaled bronchodilator and IV or rectal aminophylline, as well as a middle-aged asthmatic who remains incapacitated after an infection in spite of antibiotics and steroids.

Assessment

Severity is gauged as described in Table 3. A chest radiograph should be taken early to exclude a pneumothorax. Progress is monitored by repeated measurements of peak flow, pulse rate and arterial blood gases.

Treatment

If in doubt, status asthmaticus should be overtreated.

Bronchodilator. Aminophylline 250 mg IV is given slowly and followed by an infusion of 1 mg/kg/hr. This is usually continued for 24 hours, but occasionally is needed for longer.

Salbutamol is inhaled from a nebulizer, 2 to 4 mg four-hourly. Alternatively, salbutamol can be given intravenously 5 to 10 μg/min in place of aminophylline; there is no striking difference between the two drugs given in this way.

Adrenaline 0.5 ml 1:1,000 subcutaneously is particularly useful to cover the period before the IV drugs can be given. Terbutaline 0.25 to 0.5 mg can be used in the same way.

Steroids. Hydrocortisone 200 mg IV four hourly is given and prednisone 40 mg p.o. daily started at the same time. After 24 hours the hydrocortisone can be discontinued. Steroids take 4 to 6 hours to have an effect.

IV fluids. The need for rehydration is judged clinically and on haemoglobin and blood urea levels.

On this regimen, the patient usually improves. The peak flow rises, the heart rate falls and the Po_2 improves within 24 to 48 hours. However, the patient is still at risk of respiratory arrest for some days. Ideally treatment should continue in hospital for a week or until the peak flow returns to normal with little diurnal variation.

Artificial ventilation. This becomes necessary if the patient continues to deteriorate in spite of the above treatment. The indications are a rising Pco_2 and exhaustion. A rising Pco_2 with no other evidence of improvement is a bad sign and if it rises above 45 mm Hg, ventilation is almost inevitable. During ventilation 10 ml normal saline should be instilled hourly down the endotracheal tube to loosen mucous plugs.

Pulmonary Eosinophilia

Definition

Pulmonary eosinophilia is defined as transient shadowing on the chest radiograph with a blood eosinophilia. It is also called PIE (pulmonary infiltrates with eosinophilia).

Pathogenesis

An allergic reaction takes place in the lung with release of eosinophilic chemotactic factors. Eosinophils are released from body stores, appearing in the blood and collecting around the site of the immune reaction. The infiltrates seen on the chest radiograph are these collections of eosinophils. The commonest allergens are fungi, drugs and parasites but in a number of patients no allergen can be found. The allergic reaction produces a range of different clinical effects. Essentially these are asthma, systemic upset with fever and malaise, and vasculitis. However, in many patients there is little illness and the pulmonary eosinophilia is transient and self-limiting.

Classification

Known Causes

Fungal allergy. The fungus involved is *Aspergillus fumigatus* or, very occasionally, *Candida albicans*. The illness is chronic with asthma and systemic upset but there may be no symptoms. Vasculitis is extremely rare. The blood eosinophil count is moderately high and IgE levels raised. Allergic bronchopulmonary aspergillosis is the commonest form of pulmonary eosinophilia in temperate climates.

Drugs. Sulphonamides, nitrofurantoin, PAS, penicillins and many others are implicated. The disorder is brief, and asthma and systemic upset are rare. Very occasionally vasculitis occurs with the development of polyarteritis nodosa. The eosinophil count is moderately raised.

Parasites. *Ascaris*, microfilaria and many others are known causes. These helminths pass through the lung during their life cycle and a few individuals develop an allergic reaction. There are no symptoms or only a mild illness with *Ascaris*; a few individuals may wheeze transiently. Microfilarial infestation (tropical eosinophilia) can produce systemic upset with cough, fever, haemoptysis and occasionally wheezing. Vasculitis does not occur. The eosinophil count is very high and IgE levels are raised. The diagnosis is confirmed by the filarial complement fixation test and the infestation responds to diethylcarbamazine.

Unknown Causes

Chronic eosinophilic pneumonia. Systemic upset is common while wheezing and vasculitis are rare. The pulmonary infiltrates are peripheral in contrast to other forms of pulmonary eosinophilia and resolve with corticosteroids. Episodes of eosinophilic pneumonia may continue for a year or two and then they usually resolve spontaneously. The eosinophil count is high and the IgE level normal.

Vasculitis. Systemic upset is common and wheezing variable. This illness merges into polyarteritis nodosa and Wegener's granulomatosis. The clues that a pulmonary eosinophilia may develop into polyarteritis are a persistently raised ESR, poor response to corticosteroids and signs of systemic vasculitis, e.g. renal failure, neuropathy, hypertension. One third of patients with polyarteritis nodosa have an initial respiratory illness and half of these have a blood eosinophilia. The respiratory illness is pneumonia in 70 per cent and asthma in 40 per cent.

Allergic Bronchopulmonary Aspergillosis

Pathogenesis

Aspergillus fumigatus is a ubiquitous saprophytic fungus. Airborne spores are widespread, especially in temperate climates, and the number of spores increases in winter. The fungus thrives in humid environments at 37 °C and so is particularly well suited to flourish in the bronchial tree. It can be isolated from the sputum of five to ten per cent of normal individuals with no evidence of fungal disease.

A few individuals develop allergy to fungal protein. Type I hypersensitivity produces asthma; there is an early reaction to a skin prick test and to bronchial challenge. When type III hypersensitivity coexists it produces allergic bronchopulmonary aspergillosis; there is an early and late (six to eight hour) reaction to skin test and bronchial challenge. The late airway reaction is probably caused by an inflammatory response to complexes of *Aspergillus* antigen and precipitating antibody in the bronchial wall. This eventually leads to bronchial wall damage and proximal bronchiectasis. Some bronchi are also narrowed by plugs of *Aspergillus* mycelia (Plate 13).

Repeated bouts lead to permanent lung damage and fibrosis, especially in the upper zones.

Clinical Features

Symptoms

Episodes of cough and wheeze typical of asthma occur. However, there is often a coexisting systemic upset with malaise and fever. Brown plugs of bronchial casts may be coughed up (Plate 14).

Signs

Hyperinflation and wheezing are obvious during an attack and there may be signs of consolidation or collapse. Between attacks there is usually no abnormality.

Investigations

Radiology

Transient lung shadows appear and resolve spontaneously over one to three weeks. Often as a shadow disappears in one place another appears elsewhere in the lungs (Figure 19). The shadows

Figure 19. *(a and b) Chest radio-graph in bronchopulmonary asper-gillosis. The fleeting shadows are accompanied by a peripheral eosinophilia. (c) The same patient nine years later. Upper zone fibrosis has developed.*

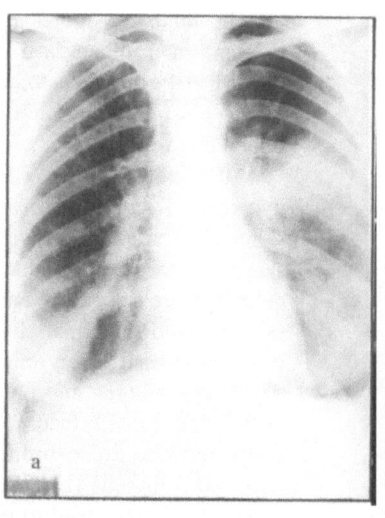

resolve within a few days of starting steroid therapy. The shadow-ing is non-segmental when eosinophils collect around a bronchus, but when *Aspergillus* plugs occlude an airway segmental col-lapse/consolidation may occur. Chronic bronchopulmonary aspergillosis produces upper zone fibrosis and contraction which may be indistinguishable from old tuberculosis.

Bronchograms show proximal segmental bronchiectasis with normal peripheral airways (Figure 20).

Lung Function Tests

Lung function tests show reversible airflow obstruction. When eosinophilic consolidation, segmental collapse or upper zone fibrosis are extensive there is a coexisting restrictive defect.

Haematology

The eosinophil count is usually 1,500 to 3,000/mm^3 during episodes of pulmonary shadowing. Between bouts and during steroid treatment the eosinophil count is normal. Occasionally a

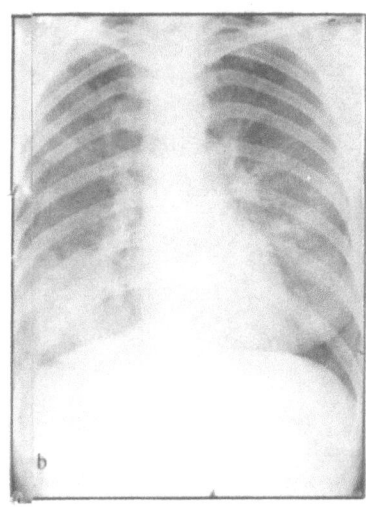
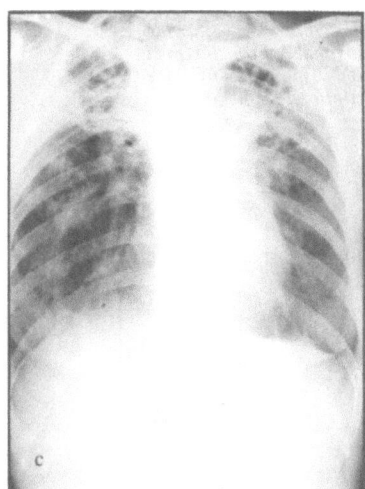

neutrophil leucocytosis is found and this suggests a bacterial pneumonia secondary to bronchial plugging and bronchiectasis.

Immunology

A positive prick test to *Aspergillus fumigatus* in a patient with pulmonary eosinophilia virtually establishes the diagnosis. When there is doubt the diagnosis can be confirmed by demonstrating precipitating antibodies to *Aspergillus* in the serum. These are present in unconcentrated serum in 70 per cent of patients and in concentrated serum in 90 per cent. Intradermal skin testing and inhalational challenge with *Aspergillus* both provoke a delayed six to eight hour reaction, but these procedures can be dangerous and are not necessary for routine diagnosis.

Treatment

Symptomatic

Sodium cromoglycate, bronchodilators and steroids are used as described above. Acute bouts require systemic steroids which

Figure 20. *Bronchogram in bronchopulmonary aspergillosis showing proximal bronchiectasis with sparing of the peripheral bronchi.*

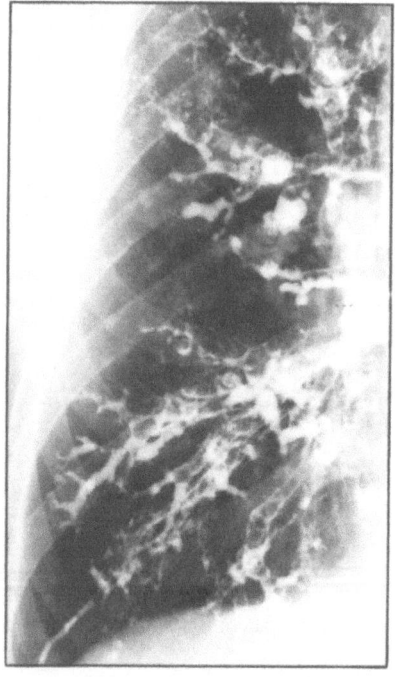

produce rapid resolution of the systemic upset and the pulmonary shadowing. Maintenance steroids are often required to control symptoms, but some patients have few acute episodes and can be maintained on inhalers alone.

Prevention of Pulmonary Damage

Repeated bouts of bronchopulmonary aspergillosis lead to bronchiectasis and upper zone fibrosis. Since the number and severity of these bouts is reduced by maintenance steroids, it is probable that they also prevent progressive pulmonary damage. Some physicians therefore prescribe maintenance steroids even when they are not necessary for controlling symptoms.

7. Rare Causes of Airflow Obstruction

The clinical and chest radiograph features of airflow obstruction are much the same whatever the cause. There is therefore a tendency to group together patients into easy diagnostic groups, such as chronic bronchitis and emphysema or asthma, or chronic obstructive lung disease. This lazy and imprecise habit can result in the rarer causes of airflow obstruction being missed altogether. The conditions discussed below are usually misdiagnosed initially—not because diagnosis is difficult, but because they are not considered.

Local Causes Affecting the Upper Airways

The site of the obstruction can be diagnosed by bronchoscopy and tomography. When the obstruction is severe enough to cause symptoms there is usually wheezing and some sputum retention. The wheeze can be heard throughout the chest and asthma is often diagnosed.

Laryngeal Palsy

Bilateral recurrent laryngeal nerve paralysis is not uncommon when malignant disease involves the mediastinum. Breathlessness and hoarseness with inspiratory stridor and a bovine cough are usually obvious but variable sputum retention with wheezing may produce attacks of breathlessness mimicking asthma. Lung function tests show airflow obstruction, but inspiratory flows are lower than expiratory. Diagnosis is by laryngoscopy, and tracheostomy relieves the obstruction.

Tracheal Stenosis

Tracheal stenosis may follow prolonged intubation or tracheostomy. When the stenosis is in the extrathoracic trachea, inspiratory stridor and low inspiratory flow rates suggest the diagnosis. Stenosis of the intrathoracic trachea is more difficult to detect clinically. Tomography or bronchoscopy are diagnostic and the treatment is surgical. Resection with re-anastomosis or insertion of a prosthesis may be necessary.

Tracheal Tumours

Carcinoma of the trachea is rare and is usually diagnosed easily when haemoptysis leads to bronchoscopy. Cylindroma of the trachea presents insidiously with breathlessness and wheeze. Occasionally fragments of the tumour are coughed up. The tumour may be seen on a penetrated chest radiograph but bronchoscopy is necessary for histology. Treatment is surgical resection.

Narrowing of the Main Bronchi

Occasionally malignant mediastinal nodes or fibrosing mediastinitis compress the bronchi sufficiently to produce symptomatic airflow obstruction. There may be a low pitched central wheeze and the narrowing is often visible on the normal chest radiograph when the bronchi are well outlined.

Emergency Treatment

When major narrowing of the large airways is severe there is a danger of asphyxia. Airflow is much improved by breathing a mixture of helium 80 per cent and oxygen 20 per cent. The low density helium has a lower turbulence than nitrogen and therefore this gas mixture flows more freely than air. The patient's breathlessness can be dramatically relieved and time gained while definitive treatment is given.

General Causes

Abnormalities of Cartilage

When bronchial or tracheal cartilage is absent or deficient, the large airways lose their rigidity. They may then collapse in expiration in the same way as the small airways. This very occasionally leads to expiratory airflow obstruction. In the Williams Campbell syndrome the cartilage is absent after the first division of the bronchi and this can lead to bronchiectasis. Occasionally the tracheal cartilage is also deficient. An acquired polychondritis produces a similar defect. All the body cartilage becomes infiltrated with inflammatory cells and loses its rigidity. This affects the nose and ears as well as airways and the diagnosis may be made by biopsy of ear cartilage.

Sarcoidosis (Plate 15)

Sarcoidosis is associated with airflow obstruction in three ways:

1. Endobronchial and peribronchiolar sarcoidosis.
2. Airway distortion from upper zone fibrosis.
3. An association with asthma.

Sarcoid granulomata can be found throughout the respiratory tract from the nose to the alveoli. Random biopsies of nasal or bronchial mucosa often show the disease in the absence of abnormal appearance or function, and detailed tests of small airway function may show mild abnormalities, insufficient to cause symptoms. More gross endobronchial sarcoid can be seen bronchoscopically as white plaques on the bronchial mucosa. These may be widespread but are particularly striking in the segmental and subsegmental bronchi.

Distortion of airways in fibrotic sarcoid may result in a mixed obstructive and restrictive pattern of lung function tests. The obstruction is not usually important and treatment is aimed at limiting the progressive fibrosis.

Asthma appears to occur slightly more often than expected in association with sarcoidosis. Treatment is along conventional lines.

Extrinsic Allergic Alveolitis with Bronchiolitis

Although the classical descriptions concentrate on the alveolitis, there is also a distinct bronchiolitis histologically. This may contribute to the breathlessness and is easily detectable on lung function testing. The importance of this is that when the bronchiolitis predominates, the chest radiograph is normal or hyperinflated, and the functional abnormality is essentially obstructive. The diagnosis may therefore be missed and an entirely preventable lung disease allowed to progress. The diagnosis may be suspected when symptoms are related to occupational exposure or contact with a pet bird or when lung function tests show airflow obstruction with a low gas transfer. The gas transfer indicates coexisting alveolitis.

Bronchiolitis

Inflammation chiefly localized to bronchioles is rare in adults, but is common in young children. The causes are viral infections (usually respiratory syncytial or adenovirus), inhalation of toxic gases (nitrogen dioxide or ammonia) or allergens (see extrinsic allergic alveolitis above).

The clinical features are distinct comprising severe breathlessness with widespread early and mid-inspiratory crackles with a normal or hyperinflated chest radiograph. Lung function tests show severe airflow obstruction, chiefly in the small airways, and air trapping with hyperinflation. The carbon monoxide gas transfer is low but the gas transfer coefficient (Kco) is normal.

Treatment is similar to that for other acute respiratory infections associated with respiratory failure, namely bronchodilators and oxygen. The role of antibiotics and corticosteroids is unproved but these should be given as they may prevent late complications. The majority of patients recover, although a few die in respiratory failure. In a minority of patients the inflammation progresses to destruction of the airways by obliterative bronchiolitis. Progressive respiratory failure may then develop some months after the initial insult. Localized obliterative bronchiolitis leads to unilateral transradiancy of the lung (McLeod's syndrome).

Rheumatoid Arthritis and Sjögren's Syndrome

An increased prevalence of airflow obstruction occurs in both of these conditions. Histology shows chronic inflammation of the small airways with some obliterative bronchiolitis (Plate 16). Although this is seldom severe enough to cause symptoms a few patients with rheumatoid arthritis have died in respiratory failure as a result of progressive airway obliteration over a few months. The cause is unknown but autoimmune inflammation and reduced defences against viral respiratory tract infections have been suggested. Patients with rheumatoid arthritis also show an increased prevalence of bronchiectasis.

Acromegaly

Acromegalics have three times the predicted mortality from respiratory disease. This is largely due to airflow obstruction which is caused by:

1. Laryngeal obstruction. The vocal cords are thickened and in some cases there is also a laryngeal myopathy. These abnormalities can be demonstrated by laryngeal tomography and confirmed bronchoscopically.

2. Small airway obstruction. Lung function tests show low flow rates at low lung volumes with a raised RV/TLC ratio, in spite of an increase in TLC. The cause of the small airway abnormality is not clear.

3. Kyphosis. Distortion of the main airways can contribute to the airflow obstruction.

All these abnormalities appear to be related to the duration of the acromegaly.

Infiltrations

Both amyloid and lymphoma may diffusely infiltrate the bronchial tree and cause obstruction. The diagnosis is made by bronchoscopy and bronchial biopsy. Lymphoma usually responds to chemotherapy. Local deposits of amyloid can be resected while generalized bronchial amyloidosis may have to be cored out via a rigid bronchoscope.

8. Respiratory Failure

Definition

Respiratory failure is defined as abnormal arterial blood gases (high P_{CO_2} or low P_{O_2}) due to a respiratory disorder. It is illogical to select arbitrary levels of blood gases at which respiratory failure begins. However, a P_{CO_2} of 49 mm Hg (6.5 Kpa) and a P_{O_2} of 60 mm Hg (8 Kpa) are usually cited.

Pathophysiology

The two basic processes causing the abnormal blood gases are failure of gas exchange and failure of ventilation. Since the causes, physiology and treatment of these two processes are quite different they must be considered separately in each patient.

Failure of Gas Exchange

The amount of air entering the lungs is adequate for respiration, but the exchange of gases between blood and inspired air is inefficient. The P_{O_2} falls because some blood passes through the lungs without being fully oxygenated. This happens in areas with low ventilation perfusion ratios. The low P_{O_2} stimulates the respiratory centre and the total ventilation increases so that more CO_2 is washed out. Increased ventilation can reduce the P_{CO_2} but cannot increase the P_{O_2} because of the difference in the haemoglobin dissociation curves for the two gases (Figure 21).

When ventilation perfusion mismatching is sufficiently severe, an increase in total ventilation cannot fully compensate. This contributes to the raised P_{CO_2} in some patients.

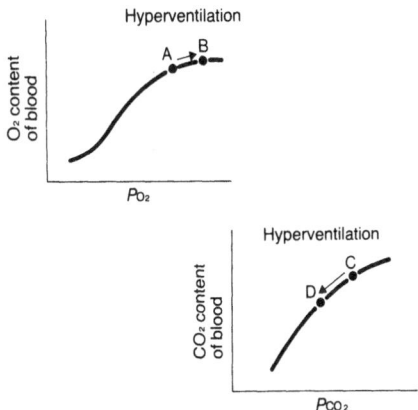

Figure 21. *Hyperventilation increases the alveolar* Po_2 *from A to B, but there is negligible increase in the* O_2 *content of blood. In contrast hyperventilation reduces the* Pco_2 *from C to D with considerable reduction in the* CO_2 *content of blood.*

The essential feature of respiratory failure due to poor gas exchange is therefore a low Po_2. The treatment is aimed at improving the Po_2 by giving supplemental oxygen. Failure of gas exchange occurs in diseases which affect the alveolus, e.g. emphysema, or the airways, e.g. asthma.

Ventilatory Failure

The situation in ventilatory failure is quite different, since the basic defect is that the total amount of air entering the lungs is inadequate for normal respiration. The Po_2 falls and the Pco_2 rises, but there is no compensatory mechanism available. Treatment must then be aimed at increasing the overall ventilation.

Ventilatory failure is caused by diminished central drive and neuromuscular disease as well as by lung disease.

Diminished ventilatory drive. This may be caused acutely by drugs (e.g. opiates, hypnotics) or intracranial disease and chronically in bronchitics by adaptation to abnormal blood gases. CO_2 narcosis itself may reduce ventilation. A rare primary defect of ventilatory drive has been described which leads to respiratory failure especially during sleep (primary alveolar hypoventilation).

Neuromuscular disorders. Respiratory failure can develop because of inadequate chest wall or diaphragmatic movement in spite of normal central drive and lungs. Muscular weakness in polyneuritis or myasthenia is usually obvious clinically but hypokalaemia and acidosis can cause weakness and contribute to ventilatory failure in chronic bronchitis. Muscular exhaustion can be important in a prolonged bout of asthma. Similarly a paralysed diaphragm, chest trauma or pleuritic pain can all limit ventilation.

Airflow obstruction. When this is very severe total alveolar ventilation is reduced and the P_{CO_2} rises. More commonly airflow obstruction contributes to the abnormal blood gases by causing ventilation perfusion mismatching and so impairing gas exchange.

In practice respiratory failure is usually due to a combination of these mechanisms.

Acute and Chronic Respiratory Failure

Many patients with chronic bronchitis have persistently abnormal blood gases. Initially the only abnormality is a low P_{O_2} due to poor gas exchange. As the obstruction increases so ventilatory failure develops and the P_{CO_2} rises. These patients are in chronic respiratory failure. The respiratory acidosis from the CO_2 retention is compensated by a metabolic alkalosis from renal retention of HCO_3. The pH is therefore normal. During acute ventilatory failure the P_{CO_2} rises and the pH falls. Renal compensation takes a few days to return the pH to normal. A low pH therefore implies acute respiratory failure.

Respiratory failure is nearly always due to diseases of airflow obstruction and the remainder of this chapter considers only these.

Clinical Features

The effects of hypoxia and hypercapnia are both seen in the central nervous and cardiovascular systems.

Hypoxia causes cerebral stimulation resulting in the patient becoming hyperactive with neuromuscular irritability. At the same time a number of cerebral functions are impaired so that incoordination, dysarthria and visual disturbances are common. Similarly higher centres are affected with loss of memory and poor concentration and disorientation and confusion are common. All these abnormalities combine to make the patient restless, noisy, uncooperative and clumsy. The heart rate increases with peripheral vasodilatation to produce a rapid bounding pulse and warm extremities.

Hypercapnia also dilates peripheral vessels and so contributes to the bounding pulse. However, the dilatation is often sufficient to cause hypotension. Sweating and peripheral pallor may result. In contrast to hypoxia, hypercapnia is a cerebral depressant and so drowsiness and precoma develop. A gross flapping tremor with inability to maintain a fixed posture is usual. The cerebral vasodilatation may cause cerebral oedema and even papilloedema, and headache, especially on waking in the morning, is common.

Investigations

Blood Gases

The diagnosis of respiratory failure is made from blood gas measurements and repeated measurements are necessary to monitor treatment. Since changes in blood gases are more important than their actual level, previous measurements done while the patient was well are particularly useful in assessing the severity of respiratory failure.

Radiology

A chest radiograph is essential to exclude precipitating factors such as pneumonia, pneumothorax or pulmonary oedema, all of which may be very difficult to diagnose clinically. However, the radiograph usually shows no recent abnormality.

Haematology and Chemical Pathology

A full blood count and blood sugar, urea and electrolyte levels should be done. The results seldom influence management but are helpful to exclude precipitating or reversible factors, such as anaemia, hypokalaemia, dehydration or diabetes. Any of these factors can cause worsening of respiratory failure and they need correction.

Bacteriology

Sputum microscopy and culture should be done and if pneumonia or a high fever are present, blood cultures taken. Only very rarely is an unexpected organism found which leads to a change in antibiotics.

Electrocardiogram

An electrocardiogram should be taken to exclude recent myocardial infarction or dysrhythmia.

Treatment

Treatment should be considered in two ways: the treatment of any reversible precipitating factor (Table 5) and the treatment of the respiratory failure itself. Oxygen is given to counteract the effects of poor gas exchange and to increase the oxygen delivered to the tissues. This is monitored by the arterial Po_2. Ventilatory failure is

Table 5. Acute respiratory failure in chronic bronchitis—precipitating factors

Acute bronchitis, pneumonia
Sputum retention
Respiratory depression (drugs, O_2)
Pneumothorax
Chest pain
Cardiac—dysrhythmia, pulmonary oedema

treated by a variety of measures aimed at improving overall ventilation and is monitored by the arterial $P\text{co}_2$.

Oxygen Therapy

Whenever the $P\text{o}_2$ is below 50 mm Hg (6.7 kPa), oxygen should be given. Patients in chronic respiratory failure with a raised $P\text{co}_2$ depend on hypoxia to stimulate the respiratory drive. When hypoxia is relieved by oxygen, the drive to ventilation is removed, overall ventilation is reduced and this leads to a dangerous rise in $P\text{co}_2$. Oxygen must be given according to the blood gas results as follows:

Low $P\text{o}_2$ with normal or low $P\text{co}_2$. Oxygen is safe and can be given by simple mask (e.g. MC or Edinburgh) 4 to 6 l/min or by nasal cannulae 4 l/min. This raises the inspired oxygen to 30 to 50 per cent. The aim is to increase the $P\text{o}_2$ to over 70 mm Hg (9.3 kPa). Often the $P\text{o}_2$ achieved will be higher, but this is perfectly safe. If the $P\text{o}_2$ remains below 50 mm Hg (6.7 kPa), either the oxygen is not being correctly given or there is severe failure of gas exchange and artificial ventilation may be needed.

Low $P\text{o}_2$ with high $P\text{co}_2$. High concentrations of oxygen may be dangerous. Oxygen should be given by 24 per cent ventimask and the blood gas measurement repeated after 15 minutes. If the $P\text{co}_2$ has risen by 10 mm Hg (1.3 kPa), or if the patient becomes more drowsy, the oxygen should be stopped. If this does not happen but the $P\text{o}_2$ remains below 50 mm Hg (6.7 kPa), the procedure is repeated with a 28 per cent ventimask, and again if necessary with a 35 per cent ventimask.

Throughout the administration of oxygen the patient should be closely observed as CO_2 retention occasionally develops over many hours.

Nurses and physiotherapists should be asked to report any increase in drowsiness or confusion. Intermittent oxygen should not be given. Theoretically this is more dangerous than continuous oxygen, and it also makes clinical observations and blood gas measurements impossible to interpret.

Improvement of Ventilation

Physiotherapy. This is the most important measure, since drowsiness and poor coughing lead to sputum retention. As well as routine physiotherapy the patient should be encouraged to cough regularly. It may be necessary for a nurse or relative to rouse the patient every hour to persuade him to bring up his sputum. When copious secretions cannot be cleared a catheter passed transnasally to the larynx can be dramatically successful in stimulating a cough and sucking away secretions. If sputum retention remains a problem artificial ventilation may be necessary. This allows access to the bronchial tree for suction and, when necessary, bronchoscopy.

Bronchodilators. Bronchospasm is seldom an important factor, but any increase in airflow may be critically valuable to the patient. Intravenous hydrocortisone and inhaled salbutamol can be given as outlined for status asthmaticus (page 67). The use of intravenous aminophylline is more controversial because of the risk of cardiac dysrhythmias.

Respiratory stimulants. The role of these remains uncertain. Nikethamide 1 mg hourly intravenously or doxapram 2 mg/min by infusion can be temporarily helpful. Unfortunately both drugs are non-specific cerebral stimulants and may provoke muscular activity or even fits. Probably they should only be used for short periods to cover a crisis, e.g. while preparing for artificial ventilation.

Artificial Ventilation

This allows control of P_{O_2} by accurate variation of inspired oxygen concentration and control of P_{CO_2} by changing the minute ventilation. There is good access to the bronchial tree to suck out secretions, and the patient can be sedated and any pain fully relieved. These advantages must be balanced against the risk of failing to get the patient off the ventilator, as well as the risks of pneumothorax and a drop in cardiac output as a result of the positive pressure.

The decision on whether or not to ventilate is difficult. It depends both on the medical condition of the patient at the time and more importantly on his quality of life over the months before admission. The medical indications are essentially deteriorating cardiorespiratory function in spite of treatment when some reversible factor is present. If there is a reasonable chance that a period of ventilation will allow recovery and a return to previous lung function, then it is indicated. The much more difficult decision is based on whether the patient's lung function was already so bad that an early death is inevitable. Some idea of the patient's life before the recent deterioration should be obtained from friends, relatives, social workers or a doctor who knew him well. If the patient was previously unable to get out or do anything for himself then ventilation is probably unkind. Ideally a decision about ventilation should be made as soon as the patient is admitted and before ventilation is actually necessary. The techniques of ventilation are beyond the scope of this book and experienced advice is essential.

Complications

Cor Pulmonale

Frusemide 40 to 120 mg IV is necessary for fluid retention. Sometimes considerable improvement in respiratory failure follows, presumably because of coexisting left ventricular failure and early pulmonary oedema. Since this can be difficult to diagnose, frusemide should be tried in resistant cases. Oxygen also improves cor pulmonale by reducing the pulmonary artery pressure and relieving myocardial hypoxia.

Gastric Bleeding

There is some evidence that regular antacids prevent this complication.

Further Reading

Chapters 1 and 2

West, J. B., *Respiratory Physiology*, Williams and Wilkins, Baltimore 1976.

West, J. B., *Respiratory Pathophysiology*, Williams and Wilkins, Baltimore, 1977.

Pride, N. B., The assessment of airflow obstruction, *Br. J. Dis. Chest* 1971, **65**, 135.

Chapters 3 and 4

Thurlbeck, W. M., *Chronic Airflow Obstruction in Lung Disease*, Saunders, Philadelphia, 1976.

Kuepers, F. and Black, L. F., Alpha$_1$ antitrypsin and its deficiency, *Am Rev. Resp. Dis.*, 1974, **110**, 176.

Chapter 5

Anderson, C. M. and Goodchild, M. C., *Cystic Fibrosis*, Blackwell Oxford, 1976.

Wood, R. E., Boat, T. F. and Doeshuk, C. F., Cystic fibrosis—the state of the art, *Am. Rev. Resp. Dis.*, 1976, **113**, 833.

Chapter 6

Clark, T. J. H. and Godfrey, S. (Eds.), *Asthma*, Chapman and Hall London, 1977.

Turner Warwick, M., On observing patterns of airflow obstruction in chronic asthma, *Br. J. Dis. Chest*, 1977, **71**, 73.

McCombs, R. P., Diseases due to immunologic reactions in the lung, *New Engl. J. Med.*, 1972, **286**, 1186.

Chapter 8

Sykes, M. K., McNicol, M. W. and Campbell, E. J. M., *Respiratory Failure*, Blackwell, Oxford, 1976.

References

Chapter 2

Webb, J. R. (Ed.), *Assessment of a Patient with Lung Disease*, Update Books, London, 1980.

Chapter 3

Fletcher, C., Peto, R., Tinker, C. and Speizer, F. E., *The Natural History of Chronic Bronchitis and Emphysema*, Oxford University Press, Oxford, 1976.

Higgins, I. T. T., *Br. Med. J.*, 1959, **1**, 325.

Mueller, R. E., Keble, D. L., Plummer, J. and Walker, S. H., *Am. Rev. Resp. Dis.* 1971, **103**, 209.

Index